Electroshock

Restoring the Mind

Max Fink, M.D.

New York   Oxford
OXFORD UNIVERSITY PRESS
1999

Oxford University Press

Oxford   New York

Athens   Auckland   Bangkok   Bogotá   Buenos Aires   Calcutta
Cape Town   Chennai   Dar es Salaam   Delhi   Florence   Hong Kong   Istanbul
Karachi   Kuala Lumpur   Madrid   Melbourne   Mexico City   Mumbai
Nairobi   Paris   São Paulo   Singapore   Taipei   Tokyo   Toronto   Warsaw

and associated companies in
Berlin   Ibadan

Copyright © 1999 by Max Fink, M.D.

Published by Oxford University Press, Inc.
198 Madison Avenue, New York, New York 10016

Library of Congress Cataloging-in-Publication Data
Fink, Max, 1923–
Electroshock: Restoring the mind / by Max Fink.
p. cm.
Includes bibliographical references and index.
ISBN 0-19-511956-8
1. Electroconvulsive therapy—Handbooks, manuals, etc.   I. Title.
RC485.F473   1999
616.89'122—DC21   98-45789

Printing (last digit): 9 8 7 6 5 4 3 2 1

Printed in the United States of America
on acid-free paper

*To Ladislas Meduna,
originator of convulsive therapy;
and
to the patients and their families
who participated freely in the studies
that established this effective treatment
for the mentally ill*

Contents

Preface

Electroconvulsive therapy is the most controversial treatment in psychiatry. The nature of the treatment itself, its history of abuse, unfavorable media presentations, compelling testimony of former patients, special attention by the legal system, uneven distribution of ECT use among practitioners and facilities, and uneven access by patients all contribute to the controversial context in which the consensus panel has approached its task.

Consensus Development Conference, 1985

Electroshock is an effective and safe treatment for those with severe mental illness. Yet many consider it so dangerous that they fear it as much as they fear the disease. The controversy is not about its efficacy or its safety, which have been proved, but about the idea that the treatment actually alters the brain, changing a person's personality and character. This mistaken perception has many roots—in the pain and complications of electroshock's early use; in the confusion with the brain-altering and ineffective treatments of insulin coma and lobotomy, which were introduced at the same time but have long been discarded; in political debates about free will and the role of the nation-state in controlling a citizen's behavior; and in fierce philosophical and economic competition among psychotherapists.

Electroshock has undergone fundamental changes since its introduction 65 years ago. It is no longer the bone-breaking, memory-modifying, fearsome treatment pictured in films. Anesthesia, controlled oxygenation, and muscle relaxation make the procedure so safe that the risks are less than those which accompany the use of several psychotropic drugs. Indeed, for the elderly, the systemically ill, and pregnant women, electroshock is a safer treatment for mental illnesses than any alternative.

Psychotropic drugs, in use during the past four decades, are the primary treatment for the mentally ill, but they are often inadequate. They may fail to relieve the disorder, or in some cases may cause side effects that are intolerable. In such instances, electroshock is certainly preferable.

Electroshock differs from other psychotropic therapies in its breadth of action. Although it was introduced as a treatment for schizophrenia, it was soon found to be equally effective in relieving the symptoms of depression and mania. And recently it has been recognized for relieving catatonia, the neuroleptic malignant syndrome, and parkinsonian rigidity. This broad applicability is confusing to clinicians who are accusto assigning certain prescriptions for specific disorders.

The trouble with these erroneous perceptions is that patients are deprived of the treatment's benefits. I have often been told about a member of a family who has been depressed for many weeks and no longer responds to the medicines that helped for a while. The patient has become worse, and the doctor now recommends electroshock. Would I answer some questions? Is that treatment still used? Is it safe? What about memory problems? What are the chances that she will get well? Why didn't the doctor suggest this in the first place? How does it work?

When distraught family members are advised to consider electroshock therapy for a relative's illness, they may suddenly recall the bizarre scenes from *One Flew Over the Cuckoo's Nest*, *The Snake Pit*, and sensational television talk shows. I will explain why the therapy is safe, effective for many mental disorders, and virtually painless.

This book contains accounts of several patients I have treated at University Hospital in Stony Brook, New York, since 1980. The adult inpatient section of the hospital admits approximately 500 psychiatric patients each year, about 50 of whom are treated with electroshock (ECT). Names and other identifying features of the patients have been changed to ensure privacy, but the treatment information is authentic.[1]

Definitions

Because convulsive therapy is a technical discipline, it has spawned its own jargon: *convulsive therapy, electroconvulsive therapy,*

ECT, electroshock, electroseizure therapy, and *EST* are accepted terms for the treatment. Some years ago, psychiatrists abandoned the word *electroshock,* in part because no shock is involved, and, more important, because it carried the connotation of pain caused by an electric contact. But because the word appears frequently in nonprofessional writings, I will use it, along with other terms.

In fact, the term *electroshock* is not accurate. When insulin was first used to treat schizophrenia, in 1933, the patients did show signs of shock: pallor, sweating, low blood pressure, rapid breathing, rapid pulse rate, and lowered levels of consciousness. Impressed with the similarity to the effects of surgical shock, practitioners called it insulin shock treatment. Seizure therapy, introduced a year later, was called convulsion treatment. A few years later, when electricity was used to induce seizures, the term *electroshock* came into use. The term *electroconvulsive treatment,* shortened to *ECT,* is a more recent coinage.

In a successful course of treatment, the brain will experience a sequence of biochemical and electrical events that are expressed in the body as epileptic *seizures.* A seizure is a coordinated brain and motor response that is present in the newborn infant, is retained throughout life, and has been observed in all animals.

Convulsion denotes an episode of muscular movements and the loss of consciousness. Neurologists refer to it as a *grand mal convulsion* or a *grand mal seizure;* other terms are *epileptic fit, epileptic convulsion, seizure,* and *fit.* In this book, I use *seizure, grand mal seizure,* and *fit* interchangeably when referring to the electrical and biochemical events in the brain that are essential for successful treatment. I use *convulsion* to refer only to the observable movements of a seizure, but since a convulsion is not necessary to successful ECT, those movements are now controlled.

A seizure induced in an animal for research purposes is called *electroconvulsive shock,* or *ECS.* In technical reports and in this book, then, ECS denotes only studies in animals; electroconvulsive therapy, ECT, and electroshock refer to the treatment of humans.

Electric shock, the actual delivery of electrical currents to the subjects, is commonly used in psychology laboratory studies of pain and sensation. At one time, such shocks were administered to patients with mental retardation to relieve their continual screaming, head banging, or self-injury, but this treatment was discarded long ago.

Acknowledgments

This book is the product of more than 45 years of interest in electroshock. I am indebted to hundreds of patients and their families, whose faith in our research efforts was evidenced by their willing consent not only to our recommended treatments but also to the vagaries, pain, and discomforts of our studies. I also thank the nurses and aides who were responsible for the daily care of these patients; without their support and faith, the clinical studies drawn upon here would not have been possible. I am indebted to my teachers—William Karliner, Lothar Kalinowsky, and Edwin A. Weinstein, all of New York, Jan-Otto Ottosson of Sweden, and Max Hamilton of England. My colleagues in studies of convulsive therapy are Martin A. Green, Robert L. Kahn, Max Pollack, Joseph Jaffe, Hyman Korin, and Donald F. Klein at Hillside Hospital; Turan M. Itil and George Ulett at the Missouri Institute of Psychiatry; Richard Abrams, Michael A. Taylor, Jan Volavka, Jiri Roubicek, Rhea Dornbush, Peter Irwin, and Donald M. Shapiro at New York Medical College; and Walter Sannita, Morton Miller, Krishnareddy Gujavarty, Larry Greenberg, Iaonnis Zervas, Georgios Petrides, Irene Carasiti, and Avi Calev at SUNY at Stony Brook. Richard D'Alli, now at the Johns Hopkins Medical School, produced our videotape. Alan Edelson, the publisher of Raven Press, encouraged me to write a textbook and to edit *Convulsive Therapy*, despite the adverse public image of electroshock.

My studies were encouraged by Israel Strauss, founder of Hillside Hospital in New York, and Joseph S. A. Miller, its medical director; Jonathan O. Cole at the National Institute of Mental Health; Alfred M. Freedman at New York Medical College; Stanley Yolles at NIMH and at SUNY at Stony Brook; Professor Dr. T. (Jack) Vossenaar in N.V. Organon of Holland; and the officers and members of the International Association for Psychiatric

Research—Arnold and Phyllis Canter, Martin and Alice Green, Theodore and Laura Israel, Henry and Maria Feiwel, Melvin and Blanche Muroff, and Donald and June Shapiro.

This volume has been edited by numerous friends; my wife, Martha; Jeffrey House of Oxford University Press; and Frances Apt of Belmont, Massachusetts, whose purple pencil did wonders in translating pedantic language into readable English.

ELECTROSHOCK

Chapter 1

∞

What Is Electroshock?

Electroshock is a treatment for severe and persistent emotional disorders. The physician, following a prescribed procedure, induces an epileptic seizure in the brain. By making sure that the patient's lungs are filled with oxygen, the physician precludes the gasping and difficult breathing that accompany a spontaneous epileptic fit. By relaxing the patient's muscles with chemicals and by inserting a mouth guard, the physician also prevents the tongue biting, fractures, and injuries that may occur in epilepsy. The physiologic functions of the body are monitored, and anything out of the ordinary is immediately treated.

The treatment is safe for patients of all ages, from children to the elderly, for people with debilitating systemic illnesses, and for pregnant women. It relieves symptoms more quickly and lastingly than the use of psychotropic drugs. Treatments are usually given three times a week for two to seven weeks. To sustain recovery, weekly or biweekly treatments are administered for several months.[1] The duration of a course of electroconvulsive therapy (ECT) is similar to that of the psychotropic medications frequently used for the same conditions.

For whom is ECT useful?

Emotional disorders may be of short or long duration; they may be manifest as a single episode or as a recurring event. Electroshock treatment is an option when the emotional disorder is acute in onset; when there are pronounced changes in mood, thought, and motor activities; when the cause is believed to be biochemical or physiological; when the condition is so severe that it interferes with the patient's daily life; or when other treatments have failed.[2]

The most recent classification system of mental disorders, published by the American Psychiatric Association in 1994, comprises more than 300 conditions. Each is defined by the symptoms presented to the physician at the time of examination and the way in which the symptoms are manifested. Mental disorders reflect persistent changes in the mind, and, except for disorders stemming from toxic or systemic illnesses, the causes are unknown. Many mental conditions, despite variations in their symptoms, can be relieved by electroshock. Among them are disorders of mood, regardless of the cause or the severity of the condition. The treatment can be of benefit to psychotic patients who are guilt-ridden or feel worthless, who believe others control their lives and influence their minds and behavior, or who are so racked by emotional pain that they contemplate suicide.

What is less well known is ECT's effectiveness in treating movement disorders by relieving the excitement and restlessness of the manic; the mutism, motor rigidity, and stupor of the catatonic; the hand-wringing of the elderly who are depressed; and the rigidity of Parkinsonism.[3] Such behavior can be altered regardless of the psychiatric classification assigned to the patient's illness (Appendix 1).

ECT is probably *not* useful for a patient with a lifelong history of mental and emotional dysfunction unless there has been an acute and well-defined onset or unless there are affective or psychotic features. Nor is it likely to help a patient with a neurosis, situational maladjustment, a personality disorder or drug dependence. If, however, such a patient evinces suicidal impulses, electroshock should be weighed as treatment (Appendix 2).

[handwritten margin note: why it doesn't work for]

When is ECT considered?

Most patients who are considered for electroshock are so ill that they are already hospitalized. They may be suffering from depression marked by suicidal threats, failure to eat, or stupor; by an excited manic state with the potential of exhaustion or self-injury; by thought disorders that threaten the lives of others; or by a catatonic stupor or excitement. Elderly patients are often referred early, especially when they suffer from a systemic illness or do not tolerate their medications.[4]

ECT is advisable when other treatments for a mental condition have failed, when normal life is severely compromised, and when medications elicit unpleasant or dangerous symptoms and their continued use is no longer feasible.

The depressed patient is usually referred for ECT after many other treatments have been tried. When he first lost interest in job and home, relatives and friends may have sought to reassure him. Perhaps they suggested a holiday. After these suggestions failed, a physician prescribed the latest antidepressant medicine or recommended formal sessions with a psychotherapist. After the patient underwent weeks or months of illness with no relief from any remedy, family members may have asked whether any other treatment was available. That is when the physician told them about electroshock.

The psychotic patient traverses much of the same ground. When a single medication fails, combinations are tried. Consideration of electroshock is delayed for the same reason that it is put off with the depressed patient: because no one realizes that electroshock can help in treating thought disorders. ECT is considered only after the patient's behavior has become so disturbing that the hospital cannot deal with it, or after the family insists on further help.

Manic and catatonic patients also endure prolonged medication trials. Referral for ECT usually does not take place until aggression, screaming, or excitement compel large doses of neuroleptic or sedative medications and continuing physical restraint.

The delay in such an effective treatment—and electroshock is that, even though patients and therapists favor medications and psychotherapy—needlessly deprives the patient. After weeks or months of illness and poor response, there is every reason to turn to electroshock.[5]

Chapter 2

∞

The Patient's Experience

With the modern technique of adequate anaesthesia and relaxant drugs
the patient loses consciousness pleasantly and quickly and is aware of
nothing until he wakes up in the recovery room. For the next couple of
hours he feels a little unsteady and ataxic; in the second series of treatments, though not in the first, I felt nausea after treatment, and on two
occasions I have vomited after reaching home by car.

A Practicing Psychiatrist, 1965

The public's images of electroshock too often reflect practices that
were discarded more than 40 years ago. The picture of a pleading
patient being dragged to a treatment room, where he is forcibly
administered electric currents as his jaw clenches, his back arches,
his body shakes, all while he is held down by burly attendants,
may be dramatic but it is wholly false. Patients are not coerced
into treatment. They may be anxious, but they come willingly to
the treatment room. They have been told why the treatment is
recommended and have given their consent.

True, the patient may be hesitant about the first treatment. He
too has seen those movies, so the procedures are explained again,
and, except for feeling a needle placed in his vein and electrodes
and measuring devices attached to his body, the patient is unaware
of the treatment as it occurs. As one patient described his treatment: "It is a nonentity, a nothing. You go to sleep, and when
you wake up, it is all over. It is easier to take than going to the
dentist."[1]

Many patients request that they be treated in the early morning so that they can return to the day's activities as soon as
possible. It is not uncommon for patients to reassure family
members about the procedure. Doctors frequently ask an experi-

enced patient to explain the procedures and the discomforts to a candidate; patients undergoing ECT have proved to be its best advocates. A practicing psychiatrist who received ECT described his experience:

> After the first treatment in both series, I felt a blunting of the acute sadness of the depression. Whereas before treatment I became tearful with very little provocation and felt intensely sad out of all proportion to the stimulus, after one single treatment I was no longer crushed by any chance sadness. The troublesome symptom of irritability also subsided early in the course of treatment.

Later, he wrote:

> I hope that this account will help to dispel the erroneous belief that E.C.T. is a terrifying form of treatment crippling in its effects on the memory and in other ways. The technique is today so refined that the patient suffers a minimum of discomfort, and the therapeutic benefits are so great in those cases where it is indicated that it is a great pity to withhold it from mistaken ideas of kindness to the patient.

Consent to treatment

A consent form, voluntarily signed by each patient, is a necessary part of electroshock treatment in the United States. The consent procedure, unique in psychiatric practice, was developed to allay fears of abuse at a time when public distrust of governmental authority had infused even the physician-patient relationship.[2] In prescribing psychotropic medications and in psychotherapy, doctors accept the patient's cooperation as evidence of consent. No written consent is required for any psychiatric treatment, even for the prescription of psychoactive drugs with well-defined risks.[3]

The consent process for ECT begins when the physician describes the benefits, procedures, risks of ECT, and alternate treatments to the patient and family. He may present a written description to the patient. Some institutions proffer an information booklet in place of the consent form; in others, a videotape explaining ECT may be shown to the patient and family.[4] When the patient agrees to treatment, he signs the consent form, under witness by a member of the medical staff and often by a family member.

Consent is given for a specified number of treatments; if more treatments are needed, the patient will be asked to renew the consent. It is not common practice to ask a patient for signed consent before each treatment, although some states do mandate this. The patient and his family members are told that the patient may discontinue treatment at any time, even before the specified number of treatments are completed. This protection clause ensures that all treatments are accepted voluntarily.

Model consent forms are available from treatment centers, in reports of the American Psychiatric Association, and in textbooks (see Appendix 3).

Involuntary treatment

Understandably, the patient wants to make the important decisions about her health care. Only when treatment is clearly necessary to preserve life will the physician or family members seek to compel it by invoking the power of the state in a court procedure.

When a patient is so ill that she requires continuing supervision to prevent self-harm, or nursing care for feeding and preventing death by inanition, state law allows a judge to mandate treatment.[5] In most states, a physician, family member, or hospital director may petition the court. In some venues, family consent is sufficient to authorize emergency treatment, as for a life-saving surgical procedure, and these rules are sometimes applied when ECT is deemed necessary.[6]

When state law has special rules for consent to electroshock, as in California and Texas, these rules of course are followed. The laws prescribe specific consent forms, procedures, and warnings, and stipulate the frequency of consent renewal. However, these elaborate procedures, devised for the protection of the mentally ill, can have detrimental consequences. They inhibit and delay the use of ECT, leading to prolonged illness and complications, including death.[7]

In most instances, when a patient refuses medical care, the physician, family, and court are unwilling to override that denial. Sadly, refusals are frequent in patients with mania or paranoia.[8]

Pretreatment examinations

Before administering anesthetics or electroshock, the physician checks the patient's history for any systemic illnesses and performs a physical examination. A complete blood count, blood chemistry tests, and an electrocardiogram (ECG) are usually done; an electroencephalogram (EEG), or detailed brain-imaging study, may be done if the physical examination suggests that such information may be useful.

The physician also examines the record of all medications that the patient has been taking; patients with heart, lung, or brain disease may regularly take medicines that could affect the quality of treatment or increase its risks. The physician can accordingly alter the medications used during electroshock. Pregnancy tests are performed in women of child-bearing age. During the first trimester of pregnancy, some medications are precluded lest they cause a structural abnormality in the fetus. A dental examination is necessary, especially for the elderly. Some dental conditions warrant the use of an individualized plastic bite, prepared by the dentist and used in each treatment. It is similar to the mouth guard used by athletes in body-contact sports. An anesthesiologist determines the patient's past experiences with anesthesia and describes the anesthesia procedures. Some anesthesiologists obtain a separate consent for this part of the treatment.

Preparation for treatment

Treatments are usually given in the morning. Because some people become nauseated by anesthetic, the patient consumes no food or liquid after midnight, which prevents vomited food from entering the lungs.

The patient usually wears a surgical gown, empties her bladder, and is then taken to the treatment room, where she lies down on a stretcher. A nurse or physician inserts a needle into a vein in her arm or foot, attaches a bag of fluid (usually sugar in water), and sets the fluid flowing at a slow rate. The intravenous line allows the easy and painless administration of anesthetics and medicines during the treatment.

Adhesive monitoring electrodes—flat disposable or reusable discs or pads to which electrical connections can be made—are applied to the skin, a painless procedure. Three electrodes are put in place for the EEG; two stimulating electrodes for the electrical stimulus; four for the ECG and heart rate; and two to measure motor movements during treatment. A recording electrode placed on the patient's finger measures the blood oxygen saturation. One blood pressure cuff on the arm measures the blood pressure; a second, placed as a tourniquet on a leg, allows the psychiatrist to observe and record the duration of the muscular signs of the seizure.[9]

The doctor or nurse explains the reasons for each connection: the ECG electrodes and blood pressure cuff permit continuous monitoring of heart rate, blood pressure, and heart rhythms; the EEG electrodes monitor the brain's electrical activity; the finger electrode and one in the ventilating mask measure oxygen saturation in the blood and the concentration of carbon dioxide in the exhaled air, assuring the anesthesiologist that the oxygen in the blood is at the correct level.

The treatment

After the preparations are completed, the patient is asked to breathe deeply as oxygen flows to a bag (about the size of a football) attached to a mask that covers her mouth and nose. Each breath takes in 100 percent oxygen instead of the 20 percent characteristic of room air, and the anesthesiologist makes sure that the oxygen flows freely during the whole treatment.

A sedative, administered through the intravenous line, puts the patient to sleep in a minute or two. Before the muscle relaxant is administered, the blood pressure cuff on the leg is inflated above the systolic blood pressure. A stimulator, applied to a nerve in the face, arm, or leg, will show whether the muscle is relaxed. When the twitches stop, the muscles are properly relaxed for the treatment.[10] The mouth guard, held in the patient's mouth by the anesthesiologist, prevents damage to the teeth or the jaw during the electrical stimulus.[11] That stimulus is then passed, and the brain seizure stimulated. The patient is not aware of the muscle relaxation, the passage of the current, the seizure, or any aspect of the actual treatment.[12]

Patient's recollections

Dr. Martha Manning, a psychotherapist, suffered from severe depression. When her illness interfered with both her professional and personal life, she consulted a psychotherapist, who prescribed antidepressants. Despite months of psychotherapy and medicine, her symptoms grew worse and she became suicidal. After half a year, her therapist suggested ECT. The journal of her experiences with depression, thoughts of suicide, and treatment with ECT was published in a book called *Undercurrents*.[13]

On the morning of her first treatment, her physician introduced her to the nurses and anesthesiologist.

> I am covered with hands. They take hold of different parts of me, staking out their territory. Voices tell me this is a dance done hundreds of times before, so I need not be afraid. But their casual confidence, their ease with my body, gives me no comfort. Just as I have lost so much of myself in the past year, now I lose more. I offer myself up to these strangers in exchange for the possibility of deliverance. Someone holds my hand and slips needles under my skin. Another slides down my gown and plants red Valentine hearts on my chest. Fingers anoint my temples with cool ointment and fasten a plastic crown tightly around my head. Wires connect me to machines that hum and beep, registering the peaks and valleys of my brain and my heart. They cover my mouth and nose with plastic and instruct me to breathe.

Dr. Manning successfully completed a course of ECT and returned to work.

Another psychologist, Dr. Norman Endler, also suffered a bout of deep depression and was plagued with suicidal thoughts. As with Dr. Manning, psychotherapy was unsuccessful. When he was given antidepressant drugs, he developed a racing and irregular heart rate, difficulty in urination, pounding headaches, nausea, vomiting, high blood pressure, and spells of weakness. After four months of failed trials, he began ECT. He described his first treatment, which he underwent as an outpatient.[14]

> I changed into my pajamas and a nurse took my vital signs (blood pressure, pulse, and temperature). The nurse and

other attendants were friendly and reassuring. I began to feel at ease. The anesthetist arrived and informed me that she was going to give me an injection. I was asked to lie down on a cot and was wheeled into the ECT room proper. It was about eight o'clock. A needle was injected into my arm and I was told to count back from 100. I got about as far as 91. The next thing I knew I was in the recovery room and it was about eight-fifteen. I was slightly groggy and tired but not confused. My memory was not impaired. I certainly knew where I was. I rested for another few minutes and was then given some cookies and coffee. Shortly after eight-thirty, I got dressed, went down the hall to fetch Beatty [his wife], and she drove me home. At home I had breakfast and then lay down for a few hours. Late in the morning I got dressed. I felt no pain, no confusion, and no agitation. I felt neither less depressed nor more depressed than I had before the ECT.

Dr. Endler recovered, returned to work, and wrote *Out of Darkness,* a popular book about his experience.

Reaction after the treatment

The patient usually breathes unassisted within three minutes after the treatment is completed. As he awakens, he is asked to give his name, date, and the name of the hospital. He may be puzzled by the questions at first, but awareness improves rapidly and his responses are usually correct within 15 minutes. After a half-hour, he is fully aware of his surroundings.

This return to awareness may vary with the patient's age and the amount of sedating medicine he has taken. Some patients are fully alert and oriented within 15 minutes, able to participate in normal daily activities. Older patients, however, may require observation for the rest of the treatment day. Some patients become agitated when they first awaken in the treatment room. The restlessness is usually controlled by an intravenous dose of Valium or Ativan.

After the treatment, the patient may be in a dreamy state, perhaps concerned about not knowing where he is or what is expected of him. Sometimes a patient complains of headache, which usually responds to aspirin or similar analgesics. If a patient has the kind of muscular soreness and stiffness that follows intensive exercise, he may get relief from an analgesic. A backache is a sign that the dose of muscle relaxant was not adequate; it can be adjusted in subsequent treatments. Occasionally, a patient will vomit when the anesthetic wears off.

Restrictions for a treatment

On the morning of a treatment, the patient uses the toilet and brushes his teeth. He takes only medicines that were prescribed for him by his physicians, and swallows them with a small sip of water. An inpatient changes to a loose gown; an outpatient comes to treatment wearing loose-fitting clothing. When the hospitalized patient returns to his room, he is encouraged to wash and dress. The elderly are supervised until it is clear that the effects of the anesthetic and the treatment have worn off. An outpatient is taken home by his caretaker.

Usually a patient's activities are not restricted, though of course he is advised to do only what he can do safely. A patient should not drive until he is completely over the effects of the anesthetic and the treatment. Again, this will take longer in older patients than in younger ones. It is up to the caretaker to watch the patient's activities and make sure that they are within his capacity.[15]

More difficult is determining when the patient is fully ready to make far-ranging decisions concerning, for example, finance, business, marriage, divorce, or the signing of wills. If such decisions cannot be deferred until the patient is well, they should be made or monitored by a responsible adult.[16]

Frequency of treatments

The schedule of treatments has been developed through experience. At first, treatments were given every three days.[17] Treatment frequency has varied from eight seizures in one day to a single seizure as an entire course.[18] Doctors at one time hoped that several seizures in a single day, under one period of anesthesia— *multiple monitored ECT* (MMECT)—would ensure clinical success without repeated use of anesthetics. But some patients still suffered memory loss, disorientation, and confusion lasting many days, without experiencing any advantages, so such schedules are not encouraged today.[19]

Daily treatments with bilateral electrode placement, known as regressive ECT, often hurt patients' orientation and memory. Patients sometimes required a few weeks of nursing care for feeding and toileting. Regressive ECT is no longer in use.[20]

Daily or twice-daily treatments are occasionally recommended for patients who are acutely delirious, excited, or suicidal, and the treatments may have an immediate good effect on suicidal tendencies and on manic delirium. But as soon as the crisis has passed, the customary treatment schedule is adopted. The current practice of two or three treatments a week, on alternate days, is effective and causes few side effects. For the elderly, two ECT treatments a week may be recommended to start with.

Treatment course

Sometimes a single treatment is successful, but that is so rare that the case is noteworthy. Almost every patient requires more treatments for a lasting beneficial effect.[21] There is no objective way, however, to predict how many treatments will be needed. The response to treatment is determined by the severity and the duration of the patient's illness, how he responds to medicine, and, most important, by the adequacy of each treatment. Doctors once thought that any seizure was beneficial, but we now know that seizures vary in their efficacy. If a fixed number of treatments is prescribed in advance, either by the psychiatrist during the consent process or by legislative fiat, as is mandated in some states, the patient may receive an inadequate number and suffer an early relapse.

Although a patient's symptoms often resolve dramatically after a few treatments, a sustained recovery requires a greater number.[22] For decades we were so concerned about the possibility of detrimental effects on memory that we restricted the treatments to the least number needed to achieve a discernable improvement. As a consequence, benefits were not sustained and the relapse rate was painfully high. Illness can recur in up to 20 percent of depressed patients within one month and in up to 50 percent within six months of a short course of treatment, even though antidepressant drugs are continued. For those with delusional depression, the relapse rates are higher.[23] Now we routinely prescribe longer courses of treatment, followed by continuation ECT or continuation pharmacotherapy. A complete course of treatment usually takes at least six months.[24]

Recovery from the illness

The depressed patient finds that with treatment her appetite and sleep return first, and then her mood improves. Agitation and restlessness disappear; suicidal preoccupations and obsessive thoughts take somewhat longer to vanish. The pace varies. The changes are most dramatic in those who have been severely ill; agitation, restlessness, strange thoughts, and preoccupations with suicide and death dissipate within the first week of treatment. The negativism, rigidity, and mutism of catatonia are usually gone after two treatments. Disorders in thought recede more slowly and require longer courses of treatment.

Recovery is a gradual process, as one feature of the illness after another recedes and the patient participates in more normal daily activities.[25] The end of a course of ECT is determined solely by the patient's clinical response. His improvement is judged according to reports of his behavior by the nursing staff and by family members, especially after he has made a home visit. When everyone agrees that the course has been helpful, then the options can be evaluated. If the patient is to continue taking a medicine, it will usually be prescribed during the last few sessions. Once continuation ECT has been recommended and an adult caretaker is on hand, the patient can be discharged from the hospital and continue treatment as an outpatient.

Continuation treatment

Most patients come to ECT after having achieved no success with prescription drugs, so it is hardly reasonable to expect the same drugs to prevent a relapse. Early reports of occasional success with psychotherapeutic medicines after ECT were confusing, but a research group discovered that many of the patients who had originally received inadequate doses got the proper kind and dosages only after successful ECT.[26]

Some depressed patients, however, come to ECT after seemingly adequate doses of appropriate medicines have had no sustained effect. In such cases, we cannot expect antidepressants to sustain the benefits of successful ECT, and we must depend on its continuation. The present experience with continuation ECT is limited, but many psychiatrists now recommend it.[27] The National Institute of Mental Health is presently supporting two large collaborative studies comparing the use of antidepressants and continuation ECT after the successful course of ECT in depressed patients.[28]

Some physicians recommend that ECT be given every other week for at least four months.[29] This schedule has been found to reduce relapse rates and improve outcomes. Weekly treatments are often too strenuous; many patients will not complete the schedule. Long-term benefits were most frequent when a biweekly schedule was maintained.

Continuation ECT is not new. Before modern psychotropic drugs were introduced in the late 1950s, most ECT patients were able to remain at home, rather than being institutionalized, having continuation ECT for months or, even years.[30] We can see that such care is not unreasonable, considering that psychotropic drugs for mental disorders are usually prescribed for years.

It is difficult to predict the number of treatments required after the initial course of ECT, but it is rarely fewer than six. Follow-up office visits with the patient and discussions with the family will determine the number. If a patient has experienced no symptoms for several months, treatment can be stopped.

Usually, depressed patients need between three and nine treatments after the successful initial course. Some may need years of weekly treatments. A woman who began ECT when she was 58 continued outpatient ECT for a decade; in all, she received more than 170 treatments.[31] Another patient, who was 31 when he began ECT for a complex form of schizophrenia, has received more than 230 treatments.[32] Such courses are unusual, but it is essential to note that halting ECT prematurely is the main cause of recurrence.

Although the administration of electroshock on an outpatient basis is not difficult, many courses have been cut short because of the inconvenience in arranging for a caretaker or the disruption in the day's activities. The highest hurdle, however, is the prejudice of family and friends who, still harboring the mistaken belief that the treatments are dangerous, dissuade the patient from further treatment with overly optimistic and premature projections of his recovery.[33]

Expected outcomes

Electroshock is prescribed for many illnesses, and various factors, especially the form and acuteness of the illness, affect the outcome. The melancholic patient with anorexia, weight loss, and insomnia of recent onset will, in almost all instances, recover within a few treatments.

But some patients with lifelong disabilities seek ECT only after months or years of ineffective treatment by other means. Many have used tranquilizers excessively or are dependent on alcohol, barbiturates, or benzodiazepines to get through a normal day and achieve some rest. Every effort is made to reduce their drug use, but the patients' dependence complicates the treatment. Patients may complain of lack of improvement and may worry about their memory and concentration, but those functions, in fact, have probably been impaired by the drugs they insist on using.

Melancholic patients with psychosis who are adequately treated have an immediate and excellent response. Unfortunately, they and their families are often so pleased by the quick relief that they discontinue the treatment, which invites relapse, often within a few weeks. The psychotic form of depression is a malignant disease that warrants extensive treatment, perhaps months of continuation ECT.

Because manic patients often come to ECT after all other treatments have failed, and after their behavior has compelled hospital care, their response to ECT may be slow. Their recovery can be sustained only by months of treatment. With those who experience a sudden onset of a manic delirium, or rapid-cycling mania, the results are excellent, provided the treatment course is intensive. Frequently, that means daily treatments.

Patients who have been psychotic for months and years may respond so slowly that the course will not show effects until they have had three to five weeks of treatment. If the illness has progressed to apathy, lack of interest, withdrawal from the family, and prolonged rumination and hallucination, the results of ECT (and other treatments) are poor.

The catatonic patient treated with electroshock almost always finds relief after two or four sessions. Absence of relief is probably the result of inadequate treatment.

Chapter 3

∞

Risks and Contraindications

Electroshock has fewer risks than does treatment with psychotropic drugs. Unlike the ingestion of medication, ECT is carried out completely under direct professional observation and control. Sixty years ago patients risked the possibility of fractures, recurrent seizures, and memory changes, but modern procedures have eliminated those risks. Fractures or recurrent seizures are rare and usually reflect technical errors. The risk of death during electroshock is one-tenth of that of women delivering spontaneous births.[1] That death from electroshock is so rare is actually surprising, given that half the patients treated with ECT are elderly and many have serious infirmities or illnesses. Our main concern is to make sure that the immediate effects of electroshock on memory and orientation do not persist.

Memory

The prevalent belief that electroshock impairs memory is based on the early experiences of patients who were treated without anesthesia or ventilation with oxygen. Such treatments were associated with severe and persistent memory losses. But present practice is no longer associated with these devastating complaints, now that careful attention is paid to oxygenation throughout the procedure and to technical features that minimize the impact of the treatments on memory. There is no longer any validity to the fear that electroshock will erase memory or make the patient unable to recall her life's important events or recognize family members or return to work. Once the patient improves, she will again be interested in her family and in social and political events, and will have the same abilities she had before she became ill.

Sometimes a patient fears that electroshock will impair the

skills that are the basis of her livelihood. That fear is groundless. It was the mental illness, not the treatment, that may have impaired her knowledge. The student who regains her normal mental state through treatment can return to her studies with the same skills she had earlier.

A few patients complain that their memories never fully return, that they have gaps in their recollection of personal history, and that memories related to work are incomplete. These patients sense an estrangement even though they can carry on their normal daily activities. They are distressed at not being able to recall the details that their friends can. But such losses are very rare.

Complaints about impaired memory

In normal life, most of us record few events of the day. Of the myriad details that impinge on our consciousness each hour of every day, few are noted clearly; even fewer are stored in our memory. The rest are permanently lost. Events that have a strong emotional component or have been orally rehearsed probably do find their place in temporary storage. When a scene is repeatedly rehearsed (think of how we learn during our schooling) or the emotional component is particularly powerful (think of family and personal events that are of great importance), the event is stored in a more permanent form, a form that permits recollection. But new experiences often overshadow earlier experiences, and, as we age, the earlier ones are crowded out. Some will be summoned up by a reminder—a photograph, a name, a sign, a melody—but most of life's daily events are lost.

When we are preoccupied by depressive and paranoid thoughts, when our moods are distorted, when we feel hopeless and helpless, when we harbor thoughts of self-harm, we register the events of our lives poorly, and few are associated with the emotional reminders that encourage recall.[2] At such times, we misinterpret the motives and statements of family members and friends, and we distort the perceptions of daily events. We are so preoccupied by the symptoms, pains, and discomforts of illness that we are vague, hesitant, and embarrassed when asked about recent events. Our responses, consequently, are slow, and we may appear so demented that our relatives fear we have Alzheimer's disease. The term *pseudodementia* has been coined to describe these conditions, which are frequently associated with an affective or psychotic disorder.[3]

Another cause of memory loss, though it is not often recognized or acknowledged, is the influence of psychotropic drugs. Almost all medications used to treat emotional disorders cause changes in brain chemistry and physiology that manifest themselves as an impairment of memory.

Anxiolytic (anti-anxiety) and sedative drugs like Valium, Xanax, Ativan, Benadryl, chloral hydrate, and barbiturates, are often given to depressed patients to improve their sleep. The effects of such drugs on orientation can last until the day after they have been taken; even a single dose may affect driving performance for 24 hours—or longer, if the dose is repeated. Tolerance to these medications (whose efficacy diminishes as the body learns how to metabolize and destroy them) develops rapidly, which encourages the use of larger doses to achieve the desired effect. Recall can then be impaired for days. This is particularly true of those sedative drugs that are discarded slowly from the body.

Lithium, used to treat manic-depressive illness, affects memory. The amount of lithium in the body is monitored to ensure an effective dosing schedule. Levels of lithium in the blood—and therefore in the brain—vary during the day and night. Immediately after the drug is ingested, the lithium level in the blood rises to the point at which it clearly impairs concentration and memory. As the hours pass, and the lithium is concentrated in the urine and discarded, the serum levels fall. The blood range effective in treatment (0.8 to 1.1 mEq/1), has only minimal effect on memory, but if the level rises above 1.3 mEq/1, the patient may become drowsy and unaware of the passing scene. These effects, which become obvious when the patient fails to drink the copious quantities of fluids needed to flush the lithium out of the body, are more frequent in the summer, when people become dehydrated with sweating. Then the serum levels rise and affect memory.

Older tricyclic antidepressants, such as Tofranil, Sinequan, and Elavil, affect concentration and memory even in proper dosages. When these drugs are given along with ECT, the combination may exaggerate the patient's confusion, perhaps causing a delirium. A transient state of confusion, disorientation, and motor excitement may occur when tissue and blood levels of antidepressant drugs become high because of accidental or intentional overdose.[4] The newer antidepressants, such as Prozac, Paxil, and Zoloft, apparently have fewer effects on memory, though reassuring data are not yet available.

Alcohol, even in small amounts, can affect memory and recall. The patient who is already taking a sedative, lithium, or an antidepressant may sustain further memory loss.

Practitioners are certainly aware of the effects of psychotropic drugs on memory. Since formal consent is not a feature of psychopharmacologic practice, however, the matter is rarely discussed, so the patient and his family are not prepared for ill effects. Everyone attributes the medicines' effects on memory to the illness. And since these medications are not only often combined with ECT, but are used as continuation treatment, their detrimental effects are often blamed solely on ECT, which then carries the full burden of the public's fear of every psychiatric treatment's cognitive effects.

Direct effect of the treatment on memory

The seizure itself, the anesthesia, the levels of oxygen in the lungs, and many technical factors of the treatment (the path of the electric currents, the frequency and number of treatments, and the form and intensity of electric currents) have direct effects on memory.[5] The effects can be severe, but our present knowledge enables the physician to provide an effective treatment with an acceptable benefit-to-risk ratio.

Because the patient was under an anesthetic during ECT, she will recall nothing that took place in the treatment room. As the anesthetic wears off, she is confused and restless. As she awakens further and recognizes the voices and faces of the doctor and the nurse, she will become calm. Soon, she will respond to her name, identify where she is, and recall the date and time of day. Disorientation about *person* is evident for 5 to 30 minutes; about *place*, an average of 10 to 40 minutes; about *time*, up to an hour. These periods are longer in older patients. When the patient returns to her room following the treatment, she will have difficulty perceiving her surroundings and recalling events for several hours. And when she is visited by her family, she may appear sleepy, vague, distant, and uninterested.

The anesthetic has both immediate and sustained effects on memory. It blots out the events of the treatment, often clouding recollection of the minutes before it was given, and persists for hours, decreasing slowly as the body sheds it. This effect of the anesthetic lasts longer in older people and in those with liver and kidney disease, for these patients get rid of the anesthetic more slowly.

Many young adults questioned immediately after ECT can recall occurrences up to the moment of anesthesia. They are able to demonstrate intellectual and performance skills—reading, writing, playing a musical instrument, planning a play in chess or bridge—soon after the treatment. Elderly patients lose such skills for hours or, in rare instances, for days.

The degree of oxygenation of the blood affects memory and recall. If the anesthesiologist has difficulty sustaining the airway or filling the lungs adequately with pure oxygen, the level in the blood and the brain may fall. When convulsive therapy was introduced, little attention was given to preserving adequate levels of oxygen, and patients sometimes stopped breathing for minutes, their blood oxygen concentrations fell, and their skin turned blue. Inadequate oxygenation of the blood led to inadequate oxygen in the brain, which could not function properly. If the anoxia lasted for many minutes, the memory suffered lasting impairment. So common were these mishaps that memory loss was considered an inevitable concomitant of successful treatment.[6] In a brilliant set of experiments, the Swedish psychiatrist Gunnar Holmberg demonstrated that electroshock given with constant high concentrations of oxygen is effective and precludes ill effects on memory.[7] By the mid-1950s, continuous oxygenation had become a standard feature of electroshock.

Individual factors affecting memory

Memory is affected by the patient's age, the duration and the severity of the illness, the presence, and seriousness of bodily disorders, and such technical factors as current intensity, electrode placement, and the frequency and number of treatments. Of these, age is the most relevant. People experience, as part of aging, the frustrating loss of recent and remote memory. The depressed elderly suffer the additional impediment of fear about their illness.

Patients often come to ECT after lengthy periods of illness—months, even years—during which fear has hindered their perception and storage of life's events. When the patients recover, often they cannot recall events that took place during their illness, especially the phase that brought them to ECT. This is true whether patients are treated by psychotherapy, by medicines, or by ECT. Because those referred for ECT are usually the most ill, and have been ill for the longest periods, the impairment of their memory is the most severe.

William Styron, in his book *Darkness Visible: A Memory of Madness*, wrote:

> But my behavior was really the result of the illness, which had progressed far enough to produce some of its most fa-mous and sinister hallmarks: confusion, failure of mental focus and lapse of memory. At a later stage my entire mind would be dominated by anarchic disconnections; as I have said, there was now something that resembled bifurcation of mood: lucidity of sorts in the early hours of the day, gath-ering murk in the afternoon and evening.... Rational thought was usually absent from my mind at such times, hence trance. I can think of no more apposite word for this state of being, a condition of helpless stupor in which cog-nition was replaced by that "positive and active anguish." ... I had now reached that phase of the disorder where all sense of hope had vanished, along with the idea of a futurity; my brain ... had become less an organ of thought than an instrument registering, minute by minute, varying degrees of its own suffering.[8]

Reports about adverse effects of ECT on memory dot the public literature. There is one from a practicing psychiatrist who received bilateral ECT in 1965, when high-energy sinusoidal currents were in use:

> Memory for recent events, during the week or so preceding treatment, appears to be the most severely affected. Mem-ories for events of several years ago seem to be impaired hardly at all.... When an event, entirely forgotten, is brought to one's notice, it sounds completely strange, for-eign and unknown. One has the feeling that a confabulation is being presented: the details of the account seem unnec-essarily elaborate, as if to make the story convincing, and the whole effect is almost laughable. Then a fragment of the

story rings true; a name is recognized, for example, and . . .
events or facts come suddenly to mind, in a linear sequence.
One is suddenly aware of a curious faculty to "feel one's
way" along this sequence, as one element leads to the next.

He describes his difficulties through an anecdote:

At the end of about two months the gaps in my memory
had been completely closed, with one amusing exception.
Several months afterwards, at a scientific meeting, I met a
psychiatrist whose face seemed very familiar, though I could
not remember his name nor where I had met him before. I
remarked on this to a friend, saying, "It must be a result of
the ECT." The friend replied, "I'm not surprised, it was he
who gave you the treatment!"[9]

After all else is said, a mental illness is a disorder of the brain,
the organ of mind and of memory. Our efforts—prescribing medicines or eliciting seizures in the brain or easing the patient's mental state by psychotherapy—are intended to change the brain's
functions. When we ameliorate a patient's symptoms, we change
the brain's ability to function properly. No one with a mental
disorder escapes alterations in memory, and electroshock is a powerful means of affecting the mind's malfunctions. Adverse effects
on memory have been minimized to the point of being undetect-
able, by any method of assessment, six weeks after completion of
treatment. In those patients who suffer estrangement more than
six weeks after treatment, there may be a recurrence of their illness, or a bad reaction to continued medicines or to a combination
of ECT and the medicines. Although improvements in our practice
have eliminated or reduced adverse effects for the many thousands
of patients treated with electroshock, they are, like all patients,
subject to the risks attendant on every form of treatment. For
those considering electroshock, the risk to memory is small compared to the benefits, and we and our patients are fortunate in
having this treatment available.

Contraindications

Are there systemic diseases that preclude the use of ECT? So much
has been learned about eliminating or minimizing risks that there

are at present no *absolute* physical or medical contraindications. Nonetheless, patients with life-threatening medical conditions are considered high-risk cases, as they would be for most anesthetic and surgical procedures.[10]

The safe treatment of a patient with recent myocardial infarction (heart attack), cerebrovascular injury (stroke), or cerebral vascular malformation does require special attention to the control of blood pressure, heart rate, and oxygenation. The presence of a growth within the skull, once thought a contraindication, is no longer considered a bar to the use of ECT. A patient with an intracranial tumor or vascular malformation can be safely treated.[11]

Pregnancy. ECT has been used safely in all stages of pregnancy; it does not precipitate miscarriage, nor does it affect the development of the fetus. When a pregnant woman suffers a severe mood disorder or psychosis, antidepressant and antipsychotic drugs are usually not prescribed, especially during the first three months of the pregnancy, because they can pass from the mother through the placenta to the circulatory system of the infant, possibly causing congenital abnormalities. For women with mental disorders during the first trimester of pregnancy, ECT is a safer treatment.

Whether medications may adversely affect the fetus in the second three months of pregnancy is unclear, so some practitioners rely on medications and some on ECT. In the final three months of pregnancy the fetus is considered fully formed, and most practitioners prefer medications. ECT is recommended when medications fail to control the illness or when the patient has had a good result with ECT in an earlier episode.

Age. ECT has been safely administered to patients as old as 102. The risks are those related to the physical deterioration associated with aging. Although the list of systemic problems of the elderly is long, none prevents the use of electroshock. Some conditions, however, make it more difficult to administer anesthetics and maintain good oxygenation, but the technical aspects of ECT are sufficiently well known that a safe treatment course can be provided. Prudence dictates, of course, elderly and systemically ill patients be treated in a hospital by skilled practitioners.[12]

For adolescents the indications, efficacy, and safety of ECT are the same as for adults.[13] The experience with ECT in prepubertal children is limited to those few cases where such conditions as catatonia or self-destructive acts were life-threatening. ECT has returned many children with acute mental disorders to normal life, but these experiences are too few to resolve doubts as to its safety.

Chapter 4

∞

Technical Features of the Treatment

The following descriptions are meant to answer questions about the techniques of treatment.

Anesthesia

The main risk of convulsive therapy in earlier decades was spine fracture. In 1952, succinylcholine, a remarkable synthetic chemical, was found to block muscle contractions.[1] When it is given intravenously it acts within a minute, and because it is rapidly destroyed by the body it is ideal for the short time needed to relax the muscles and thereby minimize any adverse effects of a convulsion.

Not only the back and jaw muscles relax, but also the muscles that control breathing. The patient under succinylcholine, then, does not breathe on his own; the breathing is monitored by an anesthesiologist or nurse-anesthetist. The patient is not aware that he is not breathing by himself, because the anesthesia blocks his awareness. Also, the duration of the anesthesia is very short. It is induced chiefly by the barbiturate Brevital, which, like the muscle relaxant, is rapidly metabolized. The period of anesthesia usually lasts three to ten minutes.[2]

Because breathing pure oxygen reduces the deleterious effects on memory, the patient receives an active and constant flow of oxygen. An open channel from the nose and mouth to the lungs is maintained by an airway tube extending from the mouth to the throat. Under certain conditions—if, for instance, the patient is obese—a tube is inserted between the mouth and the larynx to keep an open airway. The *intubation* is done after the patient is asleep and is removed before the patient wakes. Intubation, a routine procedure in general anesthesia, causes no discomfort, because the patient is unaware of it.[3]

Salivation increases, and the heart rate and blood pressure rise during treatment. A substance like Robinul or atropine, administered intravenously in the treatment room just before the anesthetic, moderates these changes. Some physicians prefer that the medication be given by intramuscular injection about 30 minutes before the treatment.[4]

The anesthesiologist, who is present during the entire treatment, makes sure the muscles are relaxed and ventilation is adequate.

Electrical energy

Modern electroshock uses a square-wave form of energy, which has a slight, if any, effect on memory.[5] The frequency of the square waves varies from 30 to 70 cycles per second, with a pulse width of 0.5, 1.0, or 2.0 milliseconds. The duration of stimulation varies between 0.2 and 8.0 seconds, and delivers from 25 to 500 millicoulombs of energy.

ECT devices enable the doctor to vary the stimulus. Since the energy that is needed depends in part on the resistance of the skin, skull, and intervening tissues, the devices allow for an estimate of the resistance between the stimulating electrodes, thereby ensuring adequate and safe treatment. Amplifiers record the EEG and the ECG during the seizure, permitting the doctor to evaluate the quality of each treatment. These devices are grounded and have special circuitry that prevents the delivery of excessive energy. There is no cause to fear that the electric currents could kill a patient.[6]

The other factors that are taken into account when adjusting the energy level are the patient's age and gender, and the type, amount, and duration of medicines he takes. The energy level is always individualized.[7] We deliver more energy to older patients than to younger ones and more to men than to women. Because the threshold rise is roughly linear with age, energy-dosing tables can help in setting the level for the first treatment. Depending on the quality of the seizure, we increase or decrease the setting for successive treatments. Some practitioners determine the actual seizure threshold during the first treatment and give successive treatments at energies a fixed amount above the threshold. This method is useful when the treatment is done with unilateral electrode placement.

Electrodes

The stimulus is delivered through flat electrodes, usually one to two inches in diameter, applied either to both temples (*bilateral electrode placement*) or to one temple and the back of the head on the same side (*unilateral electrode placement*). Some doctors place the electrodes on the forehead, about three inches apart; this is *bifrontal electrode placement*. The electrodes are either pasted on the scalp or held by an elastic band. Positioning the electrode causes no pain or discomfort, and no current flows through them until the patient is asleep and all arrangements have been made for the treatment.

The placement of the electrodes does affect the outcome of the treatment. The brain has a special center for each of its functions. In right-handed individuals, the center for the control of speech and for memory is almost always on the left side of the brain, the *dominant* side. In left-handed individuals, the speech center is usually on the right side. The influence of the currents on speech and memory, then, can either be increased or minimized according to the side on which the energy is delivered. Delivery on the nondominant side lessens the effects on memory. Since dominance for speech and memory lies in the left hemisphere in more than 95 percent of the population, the unilateral electrodes are usually placed on the right side; this is *unilateral nondominant ECT*.

Unilateral ECT, however, is clinically less effective, and patients do not improve as quickly as they do with bilateral ECT. Treatments with unilateral electrode placement require special attention to energy dosing and the use of anticholinergic drugs. Because good results with bilateral ECT are more likely, it is preferred for systemically ill patients, for whom an immediate result and a minimal number of treatments are desirable. Some doctors recommend high-dose unilateral ECT in young patients, the physically healthy, and those who express concern about the possible effects on memory and cognition.[8]

Physiologic monitoring

The heart, muscles, and brain are more active than usual during a seizure. At first, the heart rate slows and then becomes more rapid. The usual rate of 68 to 78 beats per minute (bpm) rises to 110 to 130 bpm and remains elevated throughout the seizure. The rate quickly returns to normal when the seizure ends.

Blood pressure also rises during the seizure and falls when it is over. The systolic blood pressure, usually between 110 and 160 millimeters of mercury (mmHg), goes to 140 to 200 mmHg. Occasionally, the blood pressure or heart rate requires adjustment by medication and is taken care of immediately.

Blood oxygen saturation remains between 98 percent and 100 percent, carrying its maximum amount of oxygen. If the oxygen level in the blood falls, the anesthesiologist administers more frequent doses to maintain the highest concentration in the lungs.

There are three measures of seizure. The motor convulsion is observed in a lower limb and recorded in the electromyogram (EMG), a measure similar to the EEG but one that records the rhythmic changes in the muscles. The heart rate variation is observed in the ECG; the brain's electrical activity in the EEG.

Seizure durations in the body's muscles (convulsion), as measured by the EMG, range from 20 to 60 seconds. The heart rate and EEG changes usually last longer, varying from 25 to 100 seconds for the heart rate and 30 to 150 seconds for the EEG. If the seizure in the EEG lasts for more than three minutes, longer than is needed for a good clinical effect, it is interrupted by intravenous administration of a benzodiazepine. The most effective agent for stopping a seizure is 5 to 10 mg Valium, although Ativan or Versed is also used.

An effective treatment

How can a psychiatrist judge whether a particular treatment will have the desired effect? For almost two decades, the duration of the seizure served as the index of effective treatment, with a minimum of 25 seconds for the motor seizure and at least 30 seconds in the EEG as accepted minimum standards.[9] These criteria are no longer considered rigorous. Effective treatment today requires attention to the quality of the EEG as well as the length of the seizure.[10] Seizures in duration of at least 25 seconds in the motor convulsion, 30 to 50 seconds in the heart-rate increase, and from 30 to 150 seconds in the EEG are now presumed to be effective. In the seizure EEG, we look for four distinct phases: a rapid buildup of spike activity, a prolonged period of spike and slow waves, a period of high-voltage slow waves, and an exact end point at which the electrical energy is momentarily silenced.[11]

The best clinical signs of effective treatment in the depressed patient are a rapid improvement in mood, heightened energy and appetite, a return to the usual sleep patterns, and a more normal interpersonal behavior. Unless these improve within three to five treatments, the treatment is considered weak. For the patient with thought disorder, the first changes are also those in sleep and appetite. Excitement and restlessness disappear next, and last, the patient looks on his thought disorders as strange experiences in the past.

ECT-qualified psychiatrists

Doctors who give ECT are trained first as physicians, then as psychiatrists. They usually gain their experience in ECT during their residency. When they seek additional training they enroll in a special fellowship program lasting between one and five days.[12]

A psychiatrist who intends to administer the treatment usually applies to the hospital medical board for permission to use its facilities. To obtain the privilege the physician must satisfy the institution's requirements, set according to standards suggested by the American Psychiatric Association.[13]

When a psychiatrist not trained in ECT decides that electroshock is called for, he refers the patient to a colleague who is privileged to administer it. The ECT-qualified psychiatrist assumes responsibility for the patient's care during the ECT course, returning the patient to her physician for aftercare. If continuation ECT is recommended, it is usually the joint responsibility of both therapists.

Where is treatment carried out?

Most patients receive electroshock in an ambulatory care center or in a hospital, and are allowed to go home after each treatment. Nothing in the administration of ECT necessitates that the patient remain in hospital.[14] Hospital care is encouraged, however, when the patient has a systemic illness or requires continuous nursing attention, as may be the case with the elderly or with patients subject to suicidal or homicidal preoccupations, stupor, delirium, motor excitement, or catatonia.

Not all treatment sites are equipped for a full treatment course on an ambulatory basis. Outpatient ECT calls for the treating psychiatrist to have established relationships with consulting internists, dentists, and anesthesiologists. The patient must have an adult caretaker to ensure compliance with the medication doses, to see that he takes no food before the treatment, and to protect him until the effects of anesthesia wear off. When such arrangements are difficult to provide, inpatient ECT is recommended.

ECT requires special equipment to deliver the controlled amounts of electrical energy necessary to induce a seizure, in addition to the instruments for delivering anesthesia and for monitoring seizures. In many hospitals, a treatment and recovery room suite is adjacent to, or is part of, a psychiatric inpatient treatment unit.[15]

Chapter 5

∞

Depressive Mood Disorders

Electroshock is most often used to treat disorders of mood. Mood, an internally experienced feeling, is the emotional state reflected in the way we present ourselves to others and in the ways we react to them. Mood varies with daily circumstances and is sensitive to conditions of the body, particularly physical health, hormonal activity, fatigue, and hunger.

We recognize two main disorders of mood. The first is depression, or *depressive mood disorder*, which is dominated by sadness, hopelessness, fear of the future, and persistent thoughts that life is no longer worth living. The second, called *bipolar disorder*, is dominated by feelings of grandiosity, expansiveness, increased power and energy, and excitement.[1] (Bipolar disorder is discussed in Chapter 6.)

Mood disorders may have features such as sleeplessness, delusions, pseudodementia, and catatonia. Appetite is often disrupted and weight loss may be pronounced, at times amounting to 20 percent of the body weight within a few weeks. Work, sex, and family may be disregarded. Thoughts and threats of suicide reflect the distress of a patient, who may be agitated and restless, wringing his hands and repeating phrases or sentences over and over.

The depressed patient, overwhelmed by feelings of helplessness, hopelessness, and worthlessness, dwells on thoughts of suicide. He may believe that others are watching him or talking about him; he may hear voices when no one else is present; he may be certain that his spouse is unfaithful. He may even imagine that events depicted on a television or movie screen apply directly to him. Such abnormal thoughts are *delusions;* the state of depression combined with thought disorder is labeled *delusional depression* or *psychotic depression.*

A depressed patient is commonly unaware of the day's events, registers little of what happens around him, and has a sharply compromised memory. It may be difficult for his family to distinguish his condition from dementia. When the dementia symptoms are brought about by depression, however, they can be reversed with adequate treatment. The condition is therefore known as *pseudodementia* or *reversible dementia*.

A patient may be mute; he may sit rigidly in a chair or lie motionless on his bed, unresponsive to questions and commands, seeming to be in a stupor. This state is known as *catatonia* or *depressive stupor*.

It is useful to identify these varieties of depression, because some of them call for specific treatments. Melancholic patients and those with pseudodementia often respond to antidepressant drugs, but psychotic depressed patients require high doses of antidepressant and antipsychotic medicines. Catatonic depressed patients respond to sedative drugs like the barbiturates or the benzodiazepines. Each of these disorders is responsive to electroshock. Although it is not always the first treatment of choice, it is uniformly effective, even after extended medication trials have failed.[2]

Among all current treatments for mood disorders, electroshock is the broadest and most effective. Customarily, a psychopharmacologist selects a medicine suitable for particular symptoms. He decides on different ones for the unipolar or the bipolar form of illness, for the patient with or without psychosis, and for the patient with catatonia. ECT, however, is effective for all these mood disorders.[3] Indeed, many studies find ECT to be more effective in treating mood disorders than the tricyclic antidepressants and the monoamine oxidase inhibitors.[4]

A depressive mood disorder increases the likelihood of early death, not necessarily because of suicide but because the patient's body undergoes numerous changes associated with systemic diseases like cancer and heart disease. A survey of a large urban population indicated that depressed patients were more likely to die within the one-year follow-up period than were subjects who were not depressed.[5] The finding was corroborated by a large study of patients after 10 years[6] and another study done after 16 years.[7] The rate of death during the two years after hospital treatment for a mental disorder is higher for natural and accidental causes and for suicide.[8] Higher suicide rates are not limited to patients with depression; they are reported in all psychiatric patients.[9]

Effective treatment lowers mortality rates and the incidence of suicide. Patients treated with ECT are more likely, during follow-up, to live and to demonstrate greater clinical improvement than those treated with pharmacotherapy.[10] Suicide attempts were fewer in depressed patients treated with ECT (0.8 percent) than in those treated with antidepressant medicines alone (4.2 percent).[11] Another study showed fewer suicide attempts among those in the ECT group than among patients treated with antidepressants (0 percent vs. 10 percent) or who had no history of such attempts (1.1 percent vs. 3.6 percent). Clearly, electroshock's effect on death rates among the mentally ill, particularly those with mood disorders, is an important consideration.

Case Histories

Recurrent depression

A recurrent mood disorder usually is first noticed during the patient's adolescence or early adulthood. It may develop at a time of family or personal stress, such as the death of a parent or spouse, a move from the family home, or the loss of a job. Episodes often recur when the body is under stress—in pregnancy or after the birth of a child, during menopause, or when physical changes limit the person's capacity to care for himself. Sometimes recovery is spontaneous or follows psychotherapy or drug therapy or both, but when such an intervention fails, or when the onset is rapid and intense, electroshock is the realistic option.

MARY ADAMS, a 79-year-old widow, was depressed. Her sleep and appetite were disrupted and she lost weight. She had retired after 27 years of work as a successful bookkeeper. Four years earlier her husband had died, but she remained in her apartment, caring for it and frequently visiting her two children and three grandchildren. She had lived in the community for more than three decades and had a large circle of friends.

For several months, though, her interest in friends and family had waned. She did not take care of herself and became unkempt. Although she was encouraged to visit children and grandchildren, she refused. She finally went to live in her daughter's home, where she remained in bed much of the day, thinking about her life and its failures.

She had had episodes of depression when she was 55, 72, and 77. She responded to medicine in one episode and twice to electroshock after medicines failed. In the present episode, the antidepressants Prozac, Sinequan, and Zoloft were prescribed but produced no benefit.

On her admission to the hospital she was poorly groomed, depressed, and slow in speech; she reported that she had lost 12 pounds (8 percent of her body weight) in the previous two months. Systemic examination showed that she had low blood sugar, high blood pressure, a persistently irregular heart rate, and an enlarged heart. Coumadin, Lanoxin, and Capoten were prescribed for her heart disorders, and insulin for her diabetes.

Explaining that ECT had helped her before, Mrs. Adams asked for the treatment, and she and her older daughter signed the formal consent after hearing descriptions of the possible complications. ECT was given three times the first week and twice weekly for the next two weeks.

The day after the fourth treatment Mrs. Adams's appetite returned and her self-care improved. She no longer complained of insomnia or depression. After the seventh treatment she demonstrated that she was fully oriented, recalling telephone numbers and names, and she asked to be discharged.

For five weeks, Mrs. Adams returned for outpatient ECT at weekly intervals. At the last examination her mood was normal, she had gained seven pounds, had been to the hairdresser, and was well groomed, and she talked of plans to return to her apartment and her circle of friends. After sustaining a normal mood for 14 months, however, she again became depressed and returned for additional ECT. Because of her heart disease, she was readmitted to the hospital, where she received four treatments in two weeks. She returned home and had three additional outpatient ECT. That was two years ago, and Mrs. Adams has been well since then.

Comment. While many physicians treat depression with medicine because it is less expensive than a course of ECT, electroshock may be preferred by patients who had a good response to it during a previous episode or who had observed the efficacy in others.

Patient preference is an accepted reason for ECT as treatment, without a patient's having had a prior course of medication.[12]

It would have been difficult to determine at the outset how many treatments Mrs. Adams would need. Even in an illness as responsive to electroshock as melancholic depression in the elderly, we cannot predict the necessary number of treatments. Mrs. Adams received 12 ECT for a sustained effect in the first episode, and she required seven treatments in the second. Had she been given a predetermined number of treatments—the usual number is six or eight—her treatment would surely have been evaluated as unsuccessful, and she would have been discouraged from further treatment. Reliance on a prescribed number of treatments is risky and should not be accepted by patients and their families. If not for her history of heart disease, Mrs. Adams could have been treated as an outpatient.

Delusional depression

Disorders of thought characterize severe depressive mood disorders. The combination of mood disorder and thought disorder, now recognized as a distinct clinical entity, is evident in more than half the patients hospitalized for mood disorders. A delusional depression responds infrequently to an antidepressant medicine alone; effective treatment requires one medicine for the mood disorder and another for the thought disorder. In such cases, the broad activity of ECT, which treats both aspects of the illness, makes it the preferred form of treatment.

The concept of delusional depression is relatively recent in American psychiatry. In the mid-1970s Alexander Glassman and his associates at Columbia University reported that only three of 13 delusional depressed patients (30 percent) improved, compared with 14 of 21 nondelusional patients (66 percent), when they were treated with high doses of the tricyclic antidepressant Tofranil.[13] Nine of the 10 unimproved delusional patients responded well to ECT. The authors, thinking that the presence of delusional thoughts accounted for the difference, concluded that the treatment of delusional depressed patients with only a tricyclic antidepressant would prolong suffering, lengthen the period of risk for suicide, and unnecessarily expose patients to the toxicity of the antidepressant drugs.

This study was supported by many others.[14] In one large study,

437 depressed hospital patients were treated with Tofranil in doses of 200 to 350 mg/day for 25 days or longer[15] (the dosage and duration of treatment accorded to standards for effective and adequate treatment trials). Of these, 247 (57 percent) were evaluated as recovered and were discharged. Each of the remaining unimproved 190 patients was treated with bilateral ECT, and of these, 156 (72 percent) were evaluated as recovered. In seeking to understand why 43 percent of the depressed patients had not improved with Tofranil, the authors examined these patients' psychopathological features and found that most of them were delusional.

By 1985 we knew that only a third of patients with delusional depression would recover when treated with antidepressant drugs alone and that half would recover when treated with antipsychotic drugs alone. However, two-thirds of those treated with ECT or with a combination of high doses of both antidepressant and antipsychotic drugs became well.[16]

In a two-year study of late-life depression, 47 percent of the delusional depressed patients treated with drugs relapsed earlier and more often than the nondelusional depressed (15 percent).[17] The delusional form of depression proved particularly resistant to drug therapy. The relapse rate of delusional depressed patients after successful ECT was also very high unless treatment was continued for many months.[18] Either ECT or high doses of both antidepressant and antipsychotic medicines were needed for at least half a year to sustain recovery.

Patients with the delusional form of depression are most likely to have severe abnormalities of neuroendocrine regulation, which exacerbate the bodily disturbances of the illness.[19] For this reason we have to use the most effective treatment at the earliest opportunity. Unfortunately, the recognition of this form of depression is difficult, and the frequent failure of treatment may reflect inadequate dosing for inadequate periods of time. A recent study showed that only 4 percent of delusional depressed patients had received sufficient drug treatment before being referred for ECT.[20] The common failure to recognize and adequately treat cases of delusional depression with medication (and with the rapid use of ECT) led one author to pose the question why patients with delusional depression had to sustain trials of inadequate therapies before being referred for ECT.[21]

RICHARD BURR, a 68-year-old scientist, had not graciously accepted his retirement three years earlier. A self-sufficient man, he had few friends, and his work had been the main interest in his life. He was married but had no children. Six months earlier, his wife had become bedridden, unable to manage their home.

Mr. Burr grew despondent, ate poorly, slept during much of the day, was up much of the night, bathed irregularly, complained of constipation and of abdominal, back, and neck pains, and thought that his food was poisoned. He insisted, contrary to fact, that he had heart disease and would soon die. He accused his wife of infidelity and refused to talk to her. He believed his neighbors were spying on his home, and he watched the street from behind curtained windows for hours at a time.

When he was brought to the hospital by an aide, Mr. Burr was unkempt and disheveled, walked slowly, had an unpleasant body odor, refused to answer questions, and was reluctant to let doctors examine him. He accused them of plotting to steal his money. He insisted that he was physically ill, that his condition was hopeless, and that treatment would be of no avail. At times he appeared to be hearing voices and muttering barely audible responses.

Clinical and laboratory examinations showed no signs of systemic disease other than eczema and dermatitis resulting from poor skin care. The patient's kidney functions were impaired because he had been drinking too little. Intravenous fluids and feeding were started.

He refused to take medicines, insisting that treatment was pointless because death was imminent. But his symptoms convinced the doctors that he needed immediate treatment. When they described the risks and benefits of ECT to Mr. Burr, he listened carefully, read the consent form, and then declared that he would not sign it. His wife, with whom the course of ECT was discussed, did agree to ECT for her husband's treatment. The medical director, having noted the delusional content of the patient's thoughts, the inanition and dehydration, poor self-care, and his refusal to take medicines, also recommended ECT. Although Mr. Burr refused to sign a formal consent, he allowed staff to examine him and to administer intravenous fluids, so it seemed reasonable to offer him ECT once more.[22]

The next morning he put on his pajamas and came willingly to the treatment room. Again the procedures were explained, and he was asked to move onto the stretcher. Although Mr. Burr pointed out that he had not signed the consent, he cooperated fully with instructions. An intravenous line was established, monitoring electrodes and blood pressure cuffs were applied, and anesthesia was given. During all subsequent treatments he cooperated in the same fashion. Treatments were given three times a week with bilateral electrode placement, and effective seizures were elicited. Mr. Burr soon began to drink and eat, returned to a normal sleep cycle, and showed a greater interest in his personal care. He showered when asked to, took his meals in the common room, applied the topical preparations prescribed for his skin, and drank fluids as requested. He did not, however, take the prescribed oral medicines. His delusional thoughts persisted.

After 12 treatments, Mr. Burr was no longer sure that his wife was unfaithful—indeed, he was sympathetic to her—and he was puzzled as he recollected his thoughts about the neighbors. After 15 treatments he improved enough to go home, though he was advised to continue ECT weekly for at least two months.

Mr. Burr came back for a treatment five days after his return home, but not for the second treatment. When a call to his home revealed that once again he was not eating or bathing, he voluntarily returned to the hospital to be admitted as a patient.

Eight additional treatments were given over the next three weeks. His mood improved, he gained 15 pounds, attended to his bodily care, remained puzzled by the stories of his strange thoughts, and went home to care for his wife. When he was discharged, he refused further ECT on the grounds that it was too difficult to come to the hospital for the treatments, but he agreed to take an oral medicine, so the antidepressant Zoloft was prescribed.

During a friendly exchange as Mr. Burr was leaving the hospital, he pointed out once again that he had never signed the consent for treatment. He had accepted treatment, he said, because he believed that his condition was hopeless and that he had no reason not to be a "good guy" and cooperate.

Throughout his hospitalization Mr. Burr remained fully oriented but uninterested in his wife or family. He did not read newspapers, listen to the radio, or watch television. He spent most of each day in his room, occasionally walking about the ward and taking part in communal activities when directed. After his return home, he became interested in the daily news, watched television, and read the paper. An aide was hired to take care of the house. One year later, he had maintained his weight, was sleeping well, and his illness had not recurred.

Comment. The patient's depressed mood, weight loss, insomnia, and thoughts of hopelessness, helplessness, and infidelity were signs of a delusional depression. His weight loss, dehydration, and unhealthy physical condition warranted more immediate treatment than ECT's alternatives could offer, and his improvement after 15 treatments augured well for continuation ECT. Because he discontinued the treatments, however, he quickly relapsed. The fuller course, at a regular schedule of three times per week, brought the sustained effect. Mr. Burr received 23 treatments, and his therapy was successfully continued with an antidepressant alone.

How many treatments are needed to relieve delusional depression? We cannot prescribe a fixed course, but delusional depressed patients require many more treatments than the nondelusional depressed.[23] Relapse is frequent when the treatments relieve just the symptoms and the course is short. Sustained improvement requires continuation treatment over many months.

One may question the propriety of treating a patient without a formal signed consent, but in this instance the consent by the spouse and the patient's acquiescence to treatment were considered sufficient. Mr. Burr's cooperation with the treatment and his continued voluntary compliance were evidence of consent.

Depression with pseudodementia

Some elderly people withdraw from their family and friends and lose interest in their personal care. At first they seem cantankerous and irritable, barely responding to friendly overtures. Later, they shut their doors, refuse to answer the telephone, and spend much of the day in bed. If they respond to questions, they do so slowly. Family members, fearing an Alzheimer-type dementia, arrange for the elderly person to have medical and neurological examinations. An EEG shows irregular slowing of the main frequencies, a brain CT-scan shows atrophy, or an MRI shows diffuse irregular hyperintensities, and these findings are interpreted as evidence of irreversible brain pathology. A structural dementia, usually of an Alzheimer type, is diagnosed.[24] But laboratory tests can be misinterpreted. At times, dementia of sudden onset may be the product of a depressive mood disorder. The Australian psychiatrist Leslie Kiloh described a dementia-like syndrome as a feature of a depressive mood disorder and labeled the condition *pseudodementia*.[25] The condition is hardly distinguishable from Alzheimer's disease except by a study of the history of earlier depressive episodes and a careful review of circumstances leading to the current disorder. Any time the appearance of a dementia syndrome in an adult, especially an elderly adult, is sudden and severe, the possibility of pseudodementia should be considered.[26]

To avoid errors in diagnosis the doctor must assess the history of every elderly patient with dementia for episodes of disturbed mood. Most patients are too ill to give their doctor a detailed medical history, so family members must cooperate. If there is evidence of depression, the correct diagnosis could be a mood disorder rather than dementia.

Are there risks in identifying and treating a patient who has irreversible structural brain disease as if they have pseudodementia? Suppose the patient is treated with antidepressants or ECT, but the dementia is not relieved; indeed, it grows worse. The patient will require intensive nursing care for the few weeks it will take for him to return to the pretreatment mental state, and then care should continue as before.

Suppose, however, that the patient *is* suffering from a reversible dementia, and the antidepressant treatment is effective. The patient, cured of the dementia, returns home and is again part of the family. The effort has been outstandingly worthwhile, for we have enabled the patient to reclaim her life. Such favorable odds surely argue for a course of antidepressant treatment in every elderly patient with a diagnosis of dementia, especially if the condition has made a sudden appearance. The following case is an example of such a gamble that paid off.[27]

HELEN DICKINSON, a 58-year-old married woman, was referred to our geriatric service for confirmation of the diagnosis of Alzheimer's disease. Nine years earlier, she had been depressed, sleepless, withdrawn, and had refused to eat. After being treated with the antidepressant Elavil (150 mg/day), she showed an immediate response. But two weeks later, she became confused, wandered aimlessly, and withdrew from family and friends. A computed X ray tomographic study (CT) revealed cortical atrophy, and a consulting neurologist made a diagnosis of Alzheimer's disease. The neurologist advised the family that further intervention was useless.

For those nine years, the woman's husband and their five daughters cared for her at home. Her weight dropped to 75 pounds, and she became incontinent of both bladder and bowel. Her husband retired from work to devote himself to her care and received support from his daughters and friends.

On examination, Mrs. Dickinson was thin and pale. She stared aimlessly, kept her arms wrapped around herself or moved an arm and a leg in rhythmic motions, and engaged in self-stimulatory actions, like a mechanical doll. She appeared oblivious of others in the room. As the examination progressed, her perplexity and anxiety increased. She touched paintings on the wall; she picked up magazines and glanced at them momentarily. Cognitive screening was time-consuming because her speech was slow and halting. She showed that she knew her name, but said the year was 1976 instead of 1985.

She was admitted to the inpatient psychiatric unit, and a detailed history obtained from her husband revealed previous episodes of depression. When she was 42, she had become withdrawn and noncommunicative, had lost weight, and had failed to care for herself or her family. ECT, combined with an unspecified antipsychotic medication, brought improvement. Five years later she was again withdrawn and unable to care for herself or her family. She received a second course of ECT and once more recovered. Then, when she was 49, she again became ill and was admitted to our hospital. These experiences suggested that Mrs. Dickinson's dementia was depressive in origin, not the consequence of a structural brain lesion.

Admission laboratory evaluations and a CT of the head were normal. After Mrs. Dickinson began taking the antidepressant Pamelor (75 mg/day), her appetite improved and she engaged in brief conversations. When she appeared to respond to internal auditory stimuli, the antipsychotic Haldol was added, and she received the combined treatment for three weeks. Her appetite further improved; she became continent and minimally verbal. She remained depressed, however, and electroshock was recommended. The treatments were explained to Mr. and Mrs. Dickinson and their oldest daughter. The husband and daughter both signed the consent form for ECT. With the recovery of her orientation after the fifth treatment, the treatments were explained directly to Mrs. Dickinson, and she signed the form.

After the fifth treatment, she was alert and communicative. After 13 treatments, she was fully oriented, achieved a maximum score on the cognitive Mini-Mental Test, and took care of her daily needs. She was recommended for discharge from the hospital with both ECT and Pamelor as continuation treatments.

Over the next four months, Mrs. Dickinson received ECT on average once every six days. Between treatments, she cared for herself, cooked for the family, and enjoyed her grandchildren. She traveled with her husband and attended softball games, keeping score and cheering for her favorite team.

In the following years, her symptoms returned periodically. On each occasion she became hesitant about decisions and progressively less able to work or cook. She would stand still for many minutes, staring into space; she answered questions with "I don't know," and no longer dressed herself or cared for her home. This sequence occurred over two to five days. When she was seen at these times she was withdrawn and perplexed, and she performed poorly on cognitive and memory tests. For 10 years she received 10 to 16 ambulatory treatments each year. Lithium therapy with serum levels between 0.7 and 0.9 mmol/L replaced Pamelor in the second year. The formal consent form for ECT was renewed annually, signed by both Mr. and Mrs. Dickinson. In 1995, the anticonvulsant sedative Ativan, in doses of 0.5 mg three times a day, was added to her other medications. For two years, she has remained well and has required no further ECT.

Comment. How is one to explain the abnormal CT scan at the start of Mrs. Dickinson's illness and the normal CT at the later examination? Although brain imaging by CT and MRI are said to reflect permanent characteristics of brain structure, scans sometimes do vary. The state of hydration, the position of the head for imaging, and changed exposure characteristics can alter images. In this instance, the diagnosis of Alzheimer's disease on the basis of a CT reading of cerebral atrophy was incorrect.

Over the decade during which Mrs. Dickinson received outpatient treatments, her condition was recurrent despite medication and more than 170 ECT. The features of staring, puzzlement, posturing, and mutism were prominent throughout the course of her illness, but they were not considered significant until they were recognized as characteristics of catatonia. After the benzodiazepine Ativan was prescribed in regular and large doses, she no longer required continuation ECT.[28]

Example from the literature

Jennie Forehand, a delegate to Maryland's state legislature, gives a particularly moving account of her 80-year-old mother's struggle with mental illness.[29] Her father had died after an extended illness, having spent months in intensive care, and her mother became depressed and stayed apart from family and friends. A general practitioner, finding no systemic illness, recommended that Mrs. Forehand be admitted to a home for intermediate care. There, a psychiatrist prescribed the antipsychotic Haldol, but Mrs. Forehand became restless, agitated, and withdrawn. A consultant switched her to another antipsychotic, Moban, but her behavior worsened; she became overactive and periodically incontinent. She once attempted suicide by stuffing handkerchiefs in her mouth and trying to swallow them. At another time, she ran away from the home. When she was found, wandering in the streets, she was fearful and disoriented.

She was transferred to the geriatric service at the Johns Hopkins Hospital. Because her daughter had kept an accurate account of her mother's illness and the medicines she had been given, the doctors were immediately able to consider ECT. The daughter wrote:

It was absolutely wonderful. So many people are afraid of shock treatment, but it's so different and so much better than it used to be. She had seven shock treatments. She was under anesthesia, so she felt none of it. And her memory was not impaired except that she does not remember what happened at Hopkins. A lot of people talk of that as being one of the drawbacks. But she remembers everything: past, present, everything. I have not seen any downside. . . . I think that electric shock used to be considered almost a medieval thing, just a terrible thing to do to people. And they did it in state institutions, almost as a punishment. But I am a terrific advocate for ECT because I saw the good that came from it.

When the mother was discharged, the daughter wrote:

It took her a little bit of time to adjust, but it was absolutely terrific. We stayed at my house for a couple of weeks, and then I took her back to Charlotte, because I knew the stigma of mental illness might be hard to get over. Every day we took a different group of people out to lunch to let them . . . see that she was the same self that they had known before. . . . I see people with some of these same symptoms who supposedly have Alzheimer's, but a lot of people out there tucked away, supposedly without promise, really have depression.

I don't know how you distinguish between the two, but knowing what I know now, I told my kids, "If I am ever in that situation, don't wait to try to distinguish. Just send me in for shock treatment and see if it helps." Because you don't know. I would risk it for the likelihood that it might be depression instead of Alzheimer's. Mother really lost a year of her life. And I lost a year of mine.

Depression in adolescents

The role of electroshock in the treatment of adolescents is neither well understood nor well documented. On the few occasions when ECT has been used, the results have been similar to those in adults.

For decades, psychiatrists attributed adolescent behavior disorders to faulty child rearing and family strife rather than to disorders of brain function or structure or genetics. They found fault in parental attitudes, not in the child's nervous system. This attitude focused attention on the psychological, not the biological, causes of illness, and on psychological, not biological, treatments.

The idea that adolescent behavior disorders may result as much from neurological or systemic disorders as from parental error gained ground when children with attention deficit disorder were treated successfully with stimulant drugs. In depressed adolescents, however, no benefits could be discerned after the use of most antidepressant drugs. At a 1994 conference, experts reviewed the role of ECT in the treatment of adolescents' mood disorders, and case reports of 62 patients were added to the 94 reports in previous publications.[30] Patients between 14 and 20 years of age who had major depressive syndromes, manic delirium, catatonia, or acute delusional psychoses were successfully treated with ECT, usually after other treatments had failed. There were no reports of harm to age-related faculties, such as impaired maturation, growth, or capacity to learn. On the contrary, the resolution of their mental disorders encouraged the young people to complete school and to continue their learning.[31]

Major depression in an adolescent

PETER RANDOLPH, a 16-year-old boy, was admitted to the hospital after two years of depressed mood, feelings of worthlessness and incompetence, isolation, and withdrawal from school. One year earlier he had attempted suicide with an overdose of aspirin and acetaminophen, and was hospitalized for his physical protection. He was then referred to a residential school, continued in individual psychotherapy, and took antidepressant drugs. But depression and thoughts of suicide persisted, so after numerous consultations and medications he was referred for ECT.

Mr. Randolph was a lean, well-groomed, alert young man obsessed by thoughts of helplessness, dying, and the inability to maintain his schoolwork. He had lost 40 pounds in four months (25 percent of body weight). He wanted help, but he was terrified by the thought that if ECT failed, there was no other recourse.

On the ward, he remained in his room, slept late, missed meals, and took no part in ward activities. Neuropsychological testing showed a superior intelligence quotient; on the WISC-III his verbal score was 129, his performance score was 106, and he had a full-scale IQ of 121.

After he and his parents signed the consent form he received seven treatments. Mr. Randolph rapidly lost his depressed mood and expressed interest in schooling. Throughout the course of treatment, he remained fully oriented, showed an interest in reading, and participated, with his age-related skills, in the occupational and group-therapy programs.

After returning home he received outpatient treatment twice weekly and then once a week throughout the summer. When school began, however, he again became depressed. The ECT frequency was increased to three times a week for two weeks, and his feeling of well-being returned.

Four months after his first ECT, and following 25 treatments, he showed no depression. He conscientiously took the mood stabilizer lithium and the antidepressant Nardil, and he attended weekly psychotherapy. He performed well at his normal grade level in school, acquired a girlfriend, and after a year was able to discontinue his medicines.

Comment. Mr. Randolph suffered from a major depressive mood disorder. Psychotherapy, medications, and special schooling had been ineffective. During the first ECT course and in continuation ECT, his improvement in mood and behavior was indistinguishable from that of an adult in ECT.

Mr. Randolph's parents at first had been adamantly against the use of drug therapy and ECT. Then, disheartened by the inefficacy of ongoing treatments and their son's suicidal threats, they consented to ECT, but only as a last resort. Given the success of the treatment they had most feared, the parents considered themselves fortunate to have been referred to an adolescent psychiatrist with a broad and eclectic approach.

Electroshock and prepubertal children

We have less experience with ECT in treating prepubertal children than in other age groups.[32] The earliest description of ECT in children was reported in the 1940s by the psychiatrist Lauretta Bender, at Bellevue Hospital in New York, where she treated more than a hundred children who had been hospitalized for childhood aggressivity and tantrums, suicidal acts, uncontrolled mania, and thought disorders. Many may have had structural brain disease. This was at a time before the introduction of modern psychotropic drugs, so Dr. Bender treated the uncontrollable behavior with electroshock, insulin coma, and experimental hallucinogens. ECT was helpful, but follow-up studies by others showed the benefits to be transient.[33]

The history of ECT as a treatment for children is limited to individual case reports. Psychiatrists at the University of Iowa described their experience with an 8½-year-old girl who came to them after a month of persistent low mood, tearfulness, self-depreciation, social withdrawal, and indecision.[34] She spoke in a whisper and answered questions only with prompting. Her movements were slow, and she needed help in eating and using the toilet. She repeatedly scratched her arms until she drew blood. She refused to eat. She was periodically mute, and her body would become stiff. She was bedridden much of the day and often wet the bed. The diagnosis was catatonia in a depressive mood disorder, but the psychotropic medications Paxil, Haldol, Ativan, and Pamelor were not effective.

After her parents gave their consent for a course of electroshock, she was treated in the same way an adult would have been. She soon showed greater participation in daily activities and began to feed herself. After a course of 19 treatments, she was ready to go home; the antidepressant Prozac was prescribed for aftercare. She quickly adjusted to school.[35]

At present, the use of electroshock in the treatment of prepubertal children is limited to instances of severe psychosis, catatonia, intractable depression or mania not treatable by other means.

Electroshock and the mentally retarded

The mentally retarded are prone to the same psychiatric disorders that plague the rest of the population, and they respond to the same treatments as do the mentally ill of normal intelligence. Restraints, high doses of antipsychotic drugs, and sedation are usually prescribed to treat uncontrollable outbursts and self-injury. When these fail to control behavior, electroshock is applied, with the occasional successful relief of self-injury. There is some prejudice against the use of ECT in patients with mental handicaps, and it is not limited to the public. Many psychiatrists do not administer ECT to patients under guardianship, fearing disapproval or anticipating legal difficulties for undertaking what may be perceived as a controversial treatment.

CLAUDIA SHERMAN'S development and maturation were slow, and the diagnosis of congenital mental retardation was made at an early age. When she was 12, she had temper tantrums that were associated with somnolence. An EEG showed paroxysmal activity, and the anticonvulsant Tegretol was prescribed. A psychological evaluation showed her intelligence score at 50. By the time she was 16, her tantrums, aggressivity, and periodic uncontrollable excitement warranted another EEG, which now was normal. Her behavior worsened, but lithium therapy brought about a calming effect.

When she was 19, Ms. Sherman was hospitalized for the first time; this was after four months of depressed mood, decreased appetite, and weight loss. Antidepressants and neuroleptics were added to the Tegretol and lithium, but neurotoxicity prompted doctors to replace them with the anticonvulsant Depakote. She developed severe dystonia, however, so all the medicines were discontinued.

Over the next two years Ms. Sherman was hospitalized four times, for two to five weeks each, and was treated with several new medicines, first the selective serotonin reuptake inhibitors Prozac and Zoloft, then the benzodiazepine Ativan, and then the atypical antipsychotics Clozaril and Risperdal. Although consultants and her parents considered ECT a reasonable course of treatment, and despite the pleas of her parents, who were her appointed legal guardians, no electrotherapist was willing to administer it. In February 1996, she was diagnosed as depressed and psychotic and was given Prolixin and Pamelor. Her behavior improved, but the medicines were discontinued when she again developed dystonia and urinary retention. That brought about a recurrence of the psychotic and depressive mood symptoms. Episodes of mutism and rigidity alternated with outbursts in which she would run off unless restrained. She once dived into the family swimming pool even though she was unable to swim.

When Ms. Sherman was admitted to our hospital, her family pleaded with us to consider electroshock. Their daughter, who looked her stated age of 23, would stand and stare without speaking for long periods. She would assume postures imitating others or remain in the positions to which the examiner moved her. Often she screamed and needed restraint. She appeared depressed; she refused to eat; and she remained incontinent. Her speech was unintelligible to everyone but her mother.

Brain imaging showed no definable abnormality. The EEG exhibited extensive low-voltage fast activity without spike activity or seizure-type bursts, patterns that are not epileptic but are considered the brain's response to the effects of the drugs. None of the tests supported the earlier diagnosis of epilepsy.

After the doctors arrived at a diagnosis of depressive disorder, with periodic mania and catatonia, and taking into account this patient's mental handicap, they prescribed high doses of Ativan. Although the catatonic behavior diminished, her mood symptoms, periodic excitement, and incontinence remained as before.

When the treating psychiatrist agreed to a course of ECT, both parents signed the consent form and bilateral ECT was begun. After two treatments, Ms. Sherman's mood and sleep improved, her appetite returned, she was tractable, and she responded to questions and directions. After the third treatment, all signs of catatonia were gone and her behavior was well controlled. She was discharged to her parents' home for continuation Ativan and weekly ECT. After two additional treatments, however, a holiday intervened, and she missed a treatment; she relapsed into excitement, impulsivity, and incontinence. Two treatments the following week restored her behavior. Weekly ECT sustained Ms. Sherman, and she was able to continue living at home, taking part in a daytime treatment program for patients with mental handicaps. She required no psychotropic drugs.

Comment. The syndrome of outbursts, depression, mania, and catatonia in a patient with a mental handicap does not differ from the syndrome recognized as mixed bipolar disorder in people without handicaps.[36] Psychotropic and anticonvulsant medications served Ms. Sherman well for a number of years, but her sensitivity to them precluded their continued use. Electroshock allowed her to remain at home, and her parents, grateful for the treatment, willingly described their experience in a letter to the Texas legislature when it considered banning ECT within the State.[37]

Examples from literature

Descriptions of ECT crop up in the autobiographies of several talented writers. Although the treatment is usually only a small part of their tragedy, its mention is always greeted with apprehension, often with gruesome details of the anticipated horrors. Almost always, the recommendation for ECT is rejected and other treatments are chosen. Only when all else has failed is ECT finally administered, and the narrator returns to mental health and to the community, school, or work.[38]

The psychiatrist Frederic Flach described the effects of electroshock on his daughter Rickie in the 1970s.[39] She was hospitalized when she was 14 and underwent treatment for more than a decade. After she had received three years of hospital care, intensive psychotherapy, and extensive medication, her psychiatrists recommended ECT, but the parents refused permission. Only after Rickie pleaded that something more be done for her was consent given. She received 18 treatments. Under the belief common among psychoanalysts in the 1970s that the relationship between mother and daughter had caused Rickie's illness, the therapists at the hospital restricted visits by her parents. Dr. Flach wrote:

> We hadn't seen Rickie since the treatments. . . . At my first glimpse I could not help but be startled by how womanly she looked in a rose-colored dress that Hillary [Rickie's mother] had sent for her birthday, her eyes sparkling, a bit pudgy, but on the whole a very pretty young woman.
> "How are you, sweetheart?" I asked.
> "I really feel great!"
> Hillary hugged her again. "You look so grown-up."
> "I am, Mom. Of course, my memory's not too great. In fact, I don't remember much of anything. Except for a headache every now and then, the treatments didn't hurt at all. But I must have been awful . . . I mean . . . well, Miss Henry tells me I used to behave badly and that they had to put me in isolation for a long time. Was I awful? . . . Can I go home now? Today?"

Rickie returned home, and neighbors and relatives quickly distanced themselves from mention of the illness. Talk of school and friends replaced talk of treatments. Rickie's illness recurred a few weeks after she returned to school, and the hospital doctors once again resorted to the psychotherapy and the medications that had failed before. Dr. Flach mentioned no discussion of continuation ECT. In an epilogue, Dr. Flach summarized the experience:

> Although she predictably reacted poorly to tranquilizers, such as the phenothiazines, she was repeatedly given these drugs in nearly every new treatment setting. I'll never know whether she was given an adequate course of antidepressant therapy. Her transient improvement following electric convulsive treatments remains a mystery, arguing somewhat for the presence of what psychiatrists call depression.

Although Dr. Flach was a psychiatrist, he and Rickie's therapists looked on electroshock as both a "last option" treatment and something magical. The one course of it that was administered brought about signs of recovery, but then the treatment was stopped. When Rickie relapsed, her doctors rejected further trials, claiming that the treatment had "failed." Yet the failure of psychotherapy and medication was never accepted as final. Those treatments were repeated and repeated, despite one failure after another, until the illness had run its course and Rickie returned to the community.

This true account, together with the proven safety and efficacy of electroshock, emphasizes the responsibility of child and adolescent psychiatrists to set aside the notion that the mental disorders of their patients are always due to psychological and social factors. Biological causes and biological treatments must be granted consideration. Mental disorders, like systemic disorders, do not distinguish between chronological age. Children and adolescents frequently suffer the same disorders that afflict adults, and pediatric psychiatrists should bear in mind the value of ECT for those syndromes that would call for it in the treatment of adults.

Chapter 6

∞

Manic Mood Disorders

Mania is an uncommon form of mood disorder. Those afflicted with it are overactive, intrusive, excited, and often belligerent. Many of them believe they have special powers, that they are famous or are related to famous people, and that they can read others' minds. They spend money lavishly. Voices on the radio or television are understood as direct communications. They speak rapidly, and their train of thought is often illogical and confused. They move incessantly, and sometimes write page after page of nonsense. They sleep and eat poorly, have little interest in work, friends, or family, and may require restraint or seclusion. Some are likable when in their manic state; others are angry and frightening.

Manic episodes can last for hours, days, weeks, or months. After disappearing, they may recur as repeated manic episodes, as periods of depression, or as mixed episodes of depression and mania. Such episodes are characteristic of manic-depressive illness in the older classifications. In the present classification these illnesses are identified as varieties of *bipolar disorder*, the term applied to both the manic and alternating forms. When the mood changes take place within a few days, the experience is labeled *rapid cycling*, a malignant form of the illness.

Like depression, mania is associated with disturbances in eating and sleeping, thinking, memory, and movement. The manic patient does not sleep well, eats poorly, loses weight, and has trouble concentrating on problems and planning the day's activities. His memory is impaired, often severely. Some patients are so disorganized as to appear demented and delirious.

In a particularly striking form of mania, a normal person becomes excited, restless, and sleeps poorly. He fears that neighbors are watching him, and he is easily frightened. He may hide in the house or leave it abruptly, dressed inappropriately—sometimes with no clothes—and wander about the streets. His hallucinations are vivid, and his thoughts disorganized. Confusion alternates with mutism, posturing, rigidity, and stereotyped repetitive movements. This state, identified as *delirious mania* (or *manic delirium*,) can cause physical exhaustion to the point of being a risk to life.[1] The syndrome responds quickly to electroshock.

Before electroshock, there was no effective treatment for mania. The patient was usually sedated with opioid derivatives, bromides, or chloral hydrate. Within a few years of its introduction, electroshock became the main treatment. Then Thorazine and other antipsychotic drugs were used in its place, often in heroic doses to control manic behavior.[2] Later, lithium became the standard treatment. Within the past two decades, anticonvulsant drugs have been prescribed in addition to lithium or in its stead. Even with this array of medicines some patients remain ill, and electroshock becomes the alternative.[3]

The main impediment to drug therapy or ECT in treating mania is the difficulty of obtaining consent. Because manic patients often deny their illness, they see no reason to give their agreement. Even verbal assent is not enough for ECT, because the patient must sign a consent form. The distinction between the use of medications, for which acquiescence alone is needed, and the use of ECT, for which written consent is needed, restricts the use of ECT despite its acknowledged efficacy and safety. Treatment of a patient without written consent requires an order from a state court, but obtaining the court order can be slow and expensive. Many judges refuse to order ECT in the mistaken belief that it is dangerous. As a consequence, in many venues ECT is the last resort after the failure of drug treatment, which often has been given in large doses and odd combinations.[4] It is not unusual for a manic patient to be secluded, restrained, and given heavy doses of antipsychotic medicines for weeks or months before the court order is obtained. Unfortunately, it may arrive so late that the condition has deteriorated and become a threat to life by inanition, weight loss, infection, or fever.

Case Histories

Acute manic episode
Some manic episodes develop so rapidly that they warrant hospital protection, seclusion, and physical restraint. During the patient's

periods of excitement, care must be taken to avoid his injuring himself, other patients, and the professional staff.

SARAH FRANKLIN, a 32-year-old married schoolteacher, became grandiose, intrusive, and silly. She slept poorly and was unable to conduct her classes. She spent money lavishly and claimed that God had selected her from among all women for special attention. When she was brought to the hospital emergency room by police, she laughed mischievously and spoke aloud to God. The officers had found her mumbling and singing to herself in a village mall, where she had made expensive purchases.

Mr. Franklin explained that his wife had been in this state for about three weeks. Over the past 10 years, she had shown symptoms of manic depression on and off, but her good response to lithium therapy had enabled her to continue teaching. Suddenly, a few weeks earlier, she stopped taking her medicine in the belief that she no longer needed it. When the symptoms recurred, lithium was started again and the anticonvulsant Tegretol was added. But the symptoms progressed, and hospital care was clearly necessary.

On her admission to the hospital, Mrs. Franklin was friendly; she walked around the ward, sang loudly, and insisted that she was well. She laughed inappropriately, walked into other patients' rooms, took their clothing and books, and then dropped them in the hall or in the next room. The melodies she sang were recognizable, but the words were nonsense. Her attire was gaudy, and she tried to embrace and kiss everyone she met on the ward. Her attitude was so friendly and pleasant that her audience laughed with her.

During all the medical tests she remained cooperative. Her kidney functions were intact, and the blood lithium and Tegretol levels were found to be in the clinically useful range. The lithium and Tegretol were continued, the neuroleptic Prolixin was added, and the sedative Anapsine was prescribed for those occasions when her behavior became particularly intrusive. For five days her behavior remained excited, and because she showed little response to the medications, even though her serum levels were adequate, electroshock was recommended.

The indications and risks were explained to Mr. and Mrs. Franklin together. When Mrs. Franklin joined her husband in the conference room, she danced about, singing silly ditties until her husband drew her into his lap and stroked and quieted her, allowing the discussion to continue. He viewed a videotape describing ECT, and later that day both he and she consented to the treatment.

The lithium and Tegretol were discontinued, but the Prolixin was continued. Two treatments of bilateral ECT were given the first day, and a single treatment on each of the following two days. The patient became calm and less intrusive, and by the third day she was oriented, slept through the night, and ate ravenously. At times she was incontinent of urine and recalled recent events poorly. ECT was continued on alternate days for nine additional treatments.

After three weeks, Mrs. Franklin no longer sang or was intrusive, nor did she speak to God. She was chagrined about her purchases. Her appetite and sleep returned. She was oriented to time, date, and place, and remembered the events leading to her illness.

Lithium was again prescribed, and the Prolixin was stopped within a week. After five weeks of hospital care, she was discharged to aftercare on maintenance lithium therapy. One month later she returned to work, and at the follow-up visit after 18 months she was doing well.

Comment. Mrs. Franklin's case exemplifies the efficacy of electroshock in treating delirious mania even when the condition has been unresponsive to drug therapy. When ECT is considered, lithium and anticonvulsants are usually discontinued, but neuroleptics are still given if they were already part of the treatment. Most often, lithium is discontinued before a course of ECT to avoid the possibility of a confusional syndrome, which may occur in patients with high serum lithium levels. Tegretol and other anticonvulsants are also discontinued before ECT, because their anticonvulsant effects can interfere with the production of an effective seizure.

Manic patients are treated with bilateral electrode placement, because it brings about rapid clinical effects, and the treatments are given on a daily schedule, even though such short interseizure periods may lead to confusion, disorientation, and occasional incontinence. As the time between treatments is lengthened, the confusion is quickly relieved; it is no longer present after the treatment course is completed.[5]

Recurrent angry mania with psychosis

In another variety of mania, the patient is angry, irritating, and unfriendly; she relates poorly to others and is therefore shunned and isolated. Because her thoughts are disordered, she is widely misunderstood, and she herself misunderstands questions and comments. Frustration is high and constant.

Early in the course of an illness, it is difficult to distinguish between a manic disorder and schizophrenia, since delusional thoughts, hallucinations, excitement, and aggression are characteristic of both conditions. The proper diagnosis will depend on the course of the illness; bipolar patients have remissions and relapses, and those with schizophrenia remain ill.

The diagnosis of schizophrenia limits the treatment options, which are broader for cases of bipolar disorder. The principal treatment option for the schizophrenic patient is antipsychotic drugs; the patient suffering from a bipolar disorder can also be treated with lithium, anticonvulsants, and ECT. A patient has much to gain from the multiple treatment options for manic disorder and little to lose. The wise psychiatrist does not claim to distinguish between the disorders early in a patient's illness.

DAVID GATES, a single, 38-year-old high school dropout, had been hospitalized repeatedly for impulsive and destructive behavior during the preceding 20 years. He was sure that neighbors and family were watching him, and he often directed aggressive outbursts at his parents and siblings. After wandering the streets of his village mumbling to himself, kicking objects, and threatening bystanders, he was brought to a psychiatric emergency room by the police. Disheveled, argumentative, loud, and angry, he explained in a grandiose fashion that God had spoken to him. After he was sedated with an intramuscular neuroleptic, a reading of his record of previous care indicated that he had been hospitalized four times in the preceding 13 months, each time for a similar outburst.

Three weeks before the current incident, Mr. Gates had been discharged from the hospital with prescriptions for lithium, Divalproex, Tegretol, and Thorazine. But when he was admitted this time, the levels of lithium and anticonvulsants in his blood were determined to be below therapeutic levels. It turned out that he had been unable to deal with the complexity of multiple dosing of four different medicines.

Mr. Gates had been treated with antipsychotic medications

since the first episode of his illness. During that period, he had held a laboring job in construction or in a delivery service for up to two years at a time, only to be hospitalized when he became intrusive. He frequently drank beer and wine, but alcohol abuse was not a major feature of the present disturbance.

On the ward he was unkempt and angry, lashing out at his roommate when he passed too near. Sometimes he spoke in a low voice when no one was in the room. Voices, he said, were telling him that his parents were not his real parents and that God was watching over him. His mood, he claimed, was "good"; he denied being sad or depressed, and he was well oriented for time and place. Examination found his weight to be below the standard.

In light of the failed drug trials of the preceding year, the doctor recommended ECT. Surprisingly, Mr. Gates accepted the treatment, probably in the belief that nothing could harm him. Since his parents were unavailable, his brother was called, and both he and Mr. Gates signed the consent.

All medications except Thorazine were discontinued. On the sixth day of Mr. Gates's hospitalization, bilateral ECT was begun on an alternate-day schedule. The sedative Ativan was given two hours before the first treatment, and despite Mr. Gates's insistence that he did not need treatment, he came voluntarily to the treatment room.

The response to the treatments was slow. After the eighth treatment, he shaved, showered, and asked for clean clothes. His demeanor improved. After 12 treatments, he no longer seemed to be listening to voices. On a brief leave from the hospital with his brother, he acted normally, ate in a restaurant, and shopped in the local mall. Treatment with lithium was begun, and blood serum levels were maintained at 0.5 to 0.6 mEq/l, which, while not fully therapeutic, were considered adequate to maintain the patient's mental state while ECT continued.

By the sixth week, Mr. Gates was cooperative, well oriented, and less hostile, and arrangements were made for him to live in an adult home. The lithium dose was increased, Thorazine was sustained, and he was discharged. He was to receive aftercare at a community clinic, and to continue taking the two medications twice a day. He has not been hospitalized for more than two years.

Comment. A mental illness that has gone untreated for months is far more difficult to deal with than one of recent appearance.

The repeated admissions to hospital and the complex polypharmacy in Mr. Gates's record indicated that he required more intensive treatment than had been offered. ECT combined with Thorazine returned Mr. Gates to a less hostile though barely competent state, but he was able to remain in the community. Had electroshock and neuroleptics been prescribed early in the course of his psychotic illness, especially within two years of its onset, the outcome might have been better.[6]

In some of Mr. Gates's multiple hospitalizations, the diagnosis was made of a bipolar disorder with psychosis rather than of schizophrenia, and both antimanic and antipsychotic medications were prescribed. In other instances, the diagnosis was of schizophrenia, and only antipsychotic medications were given. These periods of incomplete treatment contributed to the patient's deterioration. It was the failure of a resolution, despite multiple hospitalizations, that led the doctors to decide on electroshock. Mr. Gates was granted an opportunity to undergo treatment regardless of the psychopathology, and the gamble proved successful.[7]

Mania with psychosis (delirious mania)

In clinical psychiatry, opportunities for dramatic intervention are few. Most patients come to the psychiatrist after long and complex experience with their conditions. Delirious mania, with its acute onset, rapid evolution, and life-threatening aspects, is an exception. It is highly responsive to electroshock, but failure to recognize the condition can lead to such large doses of neuroleptics that seizures or life-threatening incidents like the neuroleptic malignant syndrome, can result. Here is a case with a successful outcome.

PHILIP HAMILTON, a 17-year-old, developed an alcoholic delirium after a weekend of partying. For two weeks he stayed home, where he had episodes of excitement. He refused to go to school, slept and ate little, and closeted himself in his room, listening to rock music. By the third week Mr. Hamilton became so excited that his parents brought him to the community hospital. He was observed to be unclean and continuously talking, singing, and beating rhythms with his hands. Sedation with Ativan proved inadequate; he sometimes needed restraints. After he was given Haldol, Mr. Hamilton developed fever, altered consciousness, rigidity, elevated blood pressure, and rapid heart rate—signs of a neuro-leptic malignant syndrome. He was treated in an intensive care facility with the withdrawal of Haldol and the use of the muscle relaxant Dentrium. The acute syndrome disappeared, but the pa-tient was psychotic and manic and was therefore transferred to our academic inpatient unit.

On admission, Mr. Hamilton was agitated, confused, and in-coherent. His lucidity waxed and waned. His speech was slurred and disorganized. He talked of having strange powers; he claimed that his parents, who accompanied him and were present, were not his real parents, and that he had been selected for a spectac-ularly successful career in finance. For minutes at a time he stared past the interviewer, not answering questions. Although he seemed oriented to time, place, and person, he could not recall the names of three objects after five minutes. His ability to do nu-merical calculations was poor, and he was unaware of current events. His temperature, heart rate, and blood pressure were nor-mal.

The medicines he was taking when he came to the academic hospital were the sedatives Ativan and Klonipin, the antipsychotic Thorazine, and the mood stabilizer lithium. His serum lithium level was low: 0.5 mEq/l. His behavior periodically called for re-straint and sedation with injections of Ativan or Anapsine.

Mr. Hamilton was suffering from acute delirious mania. When ECT was recommended to his parents, they refused to give their consent, fearing that the treatment would ruin their son's ability to get a college degree and have a productive life. But after con-sidering again the many weeks that he had been ill and his life-threatening reaction to the antipsychotic medications—and after being reassured by families of patients who were at that time being treated with ECT—the parents consented. Despite his ex-citement, the patient also agreed.

All medications except lithium were discontinued. The morning after the consent was signed, Mr. Hamilton's fourth day in the hospital, he was given ECT with brief-pulse currents, bilateral electrode placement, and Ketalar/Anectine anesthesia. An ade-quate seizure was induced, and recovery was uneventful.

Within an hour after the first treatment, Mr. Hamilton was rational and oriented, neither overactive nor delusional, and no longer in need of restraint. Later that afternoon, however, he relapsed to his manic state, and each of the next two treatments produced the same results. After the fourth treatment, however, his thoughts, mood, and affect were appropriate, his delusional ideas had disappeared, his self-care was normal, and he remained well. He was discharged after the sixth treatment with a prescription for continuation treatment with lithium and biweekly outpatient ECT. He received four additional treatments. Soon after, he returned to school and made up the work he had missed. The lithium therapy was sustained for four months, and he was then discharged from the clinic as recovered.

Comment. The syndrome of delirious mania is only occasionally recognized in patients; most of them are treated for acute psychosis or schizophrenia. When neuroleptic medicines are administered to an excited patient, especially one who has catatonic features and is dehydrated, a toxic neuroleptic malignant syndrome may develop, especially when the neuroleptic is given by intramuscular injection. Electroshock is the safer and more effective option.

Mr. Hamilton's catatonic signs were repetitive stereotyped movements, staring, and periodic negativism. Catatonic features are common in patients with mania (and depression); indeed, they occur more often in patients with mood disorders than in those with schizophrenia.[8]

Chapter 7

∞

Thought Disorders

The success of electroshock in relieving thought disorders is another of its remarkable features. Strongly held beliefs that are untrue (delusions), sensory experiences that have no basis in reality (hallucinations, illusions), and beliefs that others are paying special attention or plotting harm (paranoid thoughts) impair a person's social functioning and disrupt his family life. Such thought disorders accompany many mental disorders. They are associated mainly with schizophrenia but are also common in patients with depression, mania, toxic states, and brain disorders. Regardless of the cause or the associated signs and symptoms, ECT can relieve them.[1] This benefit is often given small notice, however, because electroshock has been widely regarded as an antidepressant treatment.

In the treatment of psychoses, the typical antipsychotic drugs Thorazine, Prolixin, Haldol, and Navane are effective in about half the cases, but relief comes slowly and dosing can be risky. Motor rigidity and tremors at one time were so frequent that dosing was based on the appearance of these motor signs.[2] Doses of the antipsychotic drugs were increased until rigidity, tremor, fixed facial expression, or slowed walking were observed. Then the doses were moved to slightly lower levels. When patients are treated in this manner for long periods, they develop persistent movement disorders—Parkinsonism (slowed shuffling gait, vacant facial expression, tremors), dystonia (persistent posturing), and dyskinesia (repetitive abnormal movements of mouth, tongue, face, and trunk). Dyskinesias occur at the rate of 4 percent per year of exposure for men and 5 percent per year of exposure for women.[3]

When the antipsychotic medications are discontinued, the psychosis so often reappears that present practice recommends they be taken for years. The new agents Clozaril, Risperdal, and Zyprexa are said not to trigger the motor rigidity and the dyskinesias, as the older drugs do.[4] But they reduce the signs of psychoses in only 30 percent of those who did not respond to the standard antipsychotic drugs.[5]

Despite these limitations, antipsychotic drugs are turned to much more often than electroshock. True, they are less expensive in time, cost, and effort. But when a drug course is ineffective, the physician may change to another medicine, combine medicines, or prescribe the latest product to come on the scene.[6] When ECT is finally considered, it is usually as a costly last resort and is almost always prescribed for too short a period.

The improvement brought about by ECT in thought disorders is slow when compared with the improvement in mood and movement disorders. The number of treatments needed is between 15 and 25, and if treatment is not continued after the patient is released from the hospital, relapse is frequent, probably within two months. A minimum course of ECT for effective relief of psychosis is one that continues for at least six months. The reluctance of psychiatrists to prescribe an adequate course and the patient's refusal to complete the recommended course are the main causes of relapse.

Antipsychotic drugs and ECT are synergistic in their effects— that is, they act in combination—so the combination is more effective than either treatment alone for physiologic reasons.[7] Antipsychotic medications reach the brain by way of the bloodstream and then penetrate into the brain cells by active transport across cell membranes. There is, however, an interface of seamless fatty membrane between the blood vessels and brain cells that prevents some substances from penetrating the cells. This interface, called the *blood-brain barrier* (BBB), prevents medications from getting to the brain cells of some patients. Physicians then must use massive doses to achieve even a minimal effect. Seizures, however, expand the spaces within the BBB, allowing the excluded molecules to cross easily.[8] It has recently been found that ECT seizures augment the effects of Clozaril in psychotic patients who are resistant to therapy.[9]

The treatment of the association of mood disorder and psychosis was described in the relief of delusional depression in Richard Burr (Chapter 5) and of mood disorder and delusional mania in the account of David Gates (Chapter 6). The following cases describe the relief of thought disorders by electroshock.

Case histories

Acute schizophrenia

When ROBERT JEFFERSON, an 18-year-old college freshman, returned home for the Christmas holidays, he did not call his high school friends; he spent most of his time alone in his room. He mumbled to himself and paid little attention to his family. While watching television, he would argue with the images on the screen and talk of his fears that the world would soon end. His appetite was not impaired, and he slept normally. A skilled piano player, he practiced for many hours but did a poor job of following the score; he introduced melodies in strange juxtapositions.

When the holidays were over, he refused to return to college, and his parents brought him to a psychiatric hospital. During the examination, he was cooperative and alert. He seemed to be listening to messages; when asked, he said his father's voice was talking to him, even though his father was not present. He could not relate the content. Although he listed his school courses and the names of his teachers, he could not recall the assignments he was to have completed over the holidays. He denied being sad or ill, yet he agreed to remain in the hospital on the advice of his parents.

Mr. and Mrs. Jefferson explained that their son's personality and behavior had changed during his final year in high school. He had not been interested in social affairs or in completing his lessons, and had played the piano continually. That summer, he stayed home instead of taking the trip he had originally planned. Since his admission to college was taken as a certainty by the family, he reluctantly set off for the campus in another city. Once there, he performed poorly.

The patient denied having used hallucinogenic drugs, and neither the urine nor blood examination showed any trace of such substances. Nor did the systemic examination turn up signs of physical illness. The diagnosis of paranoid schizophrenia was finally made, and the family was told of the treatment options— neuroleptic drugs or electroshock. The risks, benefits, and potential rate of improvement with each course were described, and the patient and the parents signed the consent form for ECT.

After the eighth treatment in a course of right unilateral ECT, Mr. Jefferson began to participate in ward activities and to play pleasant piano pieces for other patients and visitors. After he had had 11 treatments, he went home. For the remainder of the semester he lived at home and had psychotherapy twice a week. During the summer, he completed his freshman course requirements and in the fall returned to college. Within the next three years, he performed all the work for his bachelor's degree and then moved to New York City, where he composed popular music. Over the past seven years, there have been no signs of recurrence.

Comment. Robert Jefferson suffered from acute schizophrenia. The successful treatment with convulsive therapy of such acute illnesses during the first two years of symptoms was first reported by Ladislas Meduna in 1937. Such success has been repeatedly confirmed.

For the patients with an acute onset of a psychosis, antipsychotic drugs are frequently effective. A prudent treatment course should last at least six months, with an anticipated success rate of approximately 50 percent. The success rate with ECT is considerably higher. The risks of each treatment, comparable in severity and incidence, are different. Antipsychotic drugs affect movement and can cause rigidity, tremor, dyskinesia, and akathisia; ECT affects recent memory. The response is considerably faster with ECT, and it was this aspect that influenced Robert and his parents.

Many psychiatrists are concerned that the persistence of a psychosis may leave permanent scars in the brain and in thought and behavior.[10] Since electroshock is often rapidly effective in treating acute psychosis, one should question the common attitude that every psychotic patient first be treated with neuroleptic medications. And if the initial drug treatment is ineffective after six to eight weeks, it seems more reasonable to try electroshock than to prescribe another antipsychotic medicine. Unfortunately, few psychotic patients are given the option of electroshock in place of the next, and the next, antipsychotic medicine trial.[11]

Chronic schizophrenia

Five forms of schizophrenia are recognized—paranoid, catatonic, disorganized, residual, and undifferentiated. Delusions and hallucinations are prominent in the paranoid form; rigidity, mutism, negativism, and posturing are dominant in the catatonic. They are considered the *positive* signs of the illness, and patients with these signs respond to ECT. Patients suffering from the disorganized, residual, and undifferentiated forms are marked by apathy, lack of volition, a flat affect, disorganized thoughts, and limited interest in self-care and the events around them. These, the *negative* signs of the illness, develop after months and years of illness. ECT is not helpful in treating the full-blown negative form of the illness. Those patients who evince a mixture of the positive and negative signs may benefit from ECT.

STEVEN HANCOCK, 31, had been hospitalized 22 times from the time he was 18 for delusional thoughts, hallucinations, excitement, and the inability to care for himself. He first became ill during his second year at college and had some transient improvement from antipsychotic drugs. At various times he had been given several classes of medicines, including antidepressants, anticonvulsants, and sedatives. During his third hospitalization, when he was 20, he responded to a course of ECT and was able to return to college for one semester. When the illness recurred, the psychiatrist concluded that ECT had failed and he did not consider it again. Over the years, his parents sought the advice of many consultants, one of whom suggested that ECT be tried once more.

On admission to our hospital, Steven—tall, bearded, and unkempt—was mumbling to himself, posturing in a crucifixion stance, and alternating between mutism and hesitant responses to inquiries. He stated that he was Jesus Christ, that the Lord spoke often to him, and that he was bringing his message to the world. Mr. Hancock was cooperative except for bathing and shaving. Psychological testing showed his intelligence quotient to be high; EEG and blood measures were normal.

Because Mr. Hancock was still dominated by delusions, hallucinations, and catatonia, ECT was recommended. The risks and possible gains were explained to him and his parents, and they all signed the consent form.

The medicines were discontinued and a course of bilateral ECT was begun. After the third treatment, he recognized his parents and asked about his sister. The mutism and posturing became less noticeable. But his psychotic symptoms persisted despite more than 18 treatments. Puzzled by his lack of response, the doctors repeated an interseizure EEG recording.[12] Since it did not show the slowing of frequencies and the increased amplitudes associated with effective ECT, we concluded that the benefits of ECT had not yet developed and continued the course.

On the day after the twenty-third treatment, Mr. Hancock showered, shaved his beard, and asked to visit a barber. He was alert, oriented, and said he had no delusional thoughts. When he was told of his statements about Jesus and God, he was surprised, though he did recall thinking of God. After a visit from his parents, he was puzzled by the date; he had lost track of the years during which his sister had graduated from college, married, and had two children.

Treatments were continued once a week, with the neuroleptic Prolixin prescribed as maintenance treatment. When preparations were made for him to return to the community, he had to face his lack of social and work skills, though he remained fully oriented for time, place, and date, and was aware of his family's activities. Because he read very little, returning to college was not an option, and he did not accept the suggestion of acquiring training in manual skills. Rather, he has remained a resident in the state-sponsored adult home, where he participates in group activities and cares for himself. Biweekly continuation ECT inhibits his delusional thoughts and mutism. Ativan at 3 to 4 mg/day is an additional treatment directed to the catatonic signs. Various medicines, including each newly discovered neuroleptic, have been tried in place of ECT, but without success. When treatments are missed he quickly relapses to mutism and fails to care for himself. For more than eight years, he has been in continuation treatment, with more than 230 recorded ECT.

Comment. When Mr. Hancock was first treated by us with ECT, we did not recognize the significance of the catatonic signs, nor did we prescribe benzodiazepines. Our later recognition of the importance of these signs led to his present regimen. Most electrotherapists would not have encouraged the combination of the sedative anticonvulsant lorazepam with ECT, but our experience with other patients after Mr. Hancock, and our later understanding of adequate treatments using EEG criteria, led us to use both treatments concurrently. Mr. Hancock's need for lorazepam called for the occasional use of the benzodiazepine antagonist flumazenil before ECT.[13]

A son with schizophrenia

The lack of support for ECT as treatment for schizophrenia is widespread. Here, in an example from 1998, a father is writing about the experience of his schizophrenic son. Peter Wyden, a writer with more than 14 books to his credit, described the travail of more than 25 years suffered by his son Jeffrey, who became ill late in adolescence.[14] He detailed his son's symptoms, which were typical of schizophrenia, and the course of his hospitalizations and extensive treatment with medications and psychotherapy. When electroshock was mentioned, the father became even more disheartened, because he had read negative accounts of it.[15]

> Still, I didn't want my squeamishness to deprive Jeff of treatment that might help him. . . . Overriding to me were Jeff's feelings about his worsening state. He was no longer questioning that he was ill. He informed me that a fellow patient had told him how much she had been helped by shock treatments and that he was convinced he needed them.
>
> I was still not convinced that the likely benefits were worth the risk of a permanent memory loss, and so [Dr.] Kaplan arranged for an evaluation of Jeff's overall status at the federal government's National Institute of Mental Health in suburban Washington. . . . The verdict on electroshock was something like a shrug of the shoulders. No one overtly opposed it.

On reading the NIMH records of his son's hospitalization, Mr. Wyden wrote:

> Regarding the usefulness of ECT, the doctors were less definitive. "It is felt that Jeffrey may benefit from a course of electro-convulsive therapy . . . [but] there is no clear indication for electro-convulsive therapy at this time."

Because Jeff Wyden was in a state hospital in California, ECT could be administered only by court order. The father wrote:

> Regrettably, the application on behalf of Jeff pushed the bureaucracy into temporary paralysis. Its medical and judicial arms were not synchronized. The hospital had withdrawn Jeff's protective medications, but the judge had not issued an OK to proceed with the treatments. In the language of

psychiatry, Jeff had "regressed" and "decompensated." In my language, he was bucking in restraints and screaming.

Finally Mr. Wyden appealed to the judge and gained permission for ECT.[16]

> Jeff was given a series of twelve shock treatments in June. The treatments were uneventful, the aftermath unexpected: electrifying, simply wonderful. His mind cleared. His spirits soared. Almost immediately, out came the "old Jeff," witty, sharp, self-assured. It was like a liberating magic trick.

But within three months, Jeff had relapsed and returned to the hospital, where he was given one medication after another.[17]

California law freely permitted physicians to administer drugs; use wrist, ankle, and body restraints; and isolate the patient in seclusion rooms. But it sent the father on tortuous paths to get court approval for a treatment that proved to be of significant clinical benefit.

Often, ECT is initially rejected for thought disorders and is tried only after a long time. It typically brings about a good clinical effect—and is then discontinued. When there is a relapse, the patient, family, and treating professionals conclude that electroshock failed. What is assumed to be a failure of electroshock in these instances is rather the failure of practitioners to consider that a patient who is seriously ill, and who may have been ill for a prolonged period, is unlikely to be cured by a treatment of short duration. Yet when psychotherapy and medications are prescribed after the supposed failure of ECT, they are kept up interminably, whether they prove beneficial or useless. No one seems to grasp the logical conclusion that had continuation ECT been prescribed, the benefits would likely have been maintained.

Chapter 8

∞

Movement Disorders

Patients with mental disorders exhibit a range of abnormal movements. Some of the severely depressed are given to hand-wringing, pacing, and restlessness. Others lie in bed, stare into space, and posture for hours or days. At times, the latter behavior is so extreme as to be defined as stupor. Psychotic patients exhibit tremors or peculiar facial and body movements described as Parkinsonism, dystonia, or dyskinesia. Manic patients are in constant motion.

Little attention is paid to such behavior unless it overwhelms the patient's life, but it does distress the patient, the family, and the community. These motor symptoms often bring psychiatric patients to medical care.

Case histories

Catatonia

The behavior characterized by muscular rigidity, unusual posturing, negativism (refusal to obey simple commands), mutism (persistent silence), echolalia (repetition of what has been said), echopraxia (imitation of movements), and stereotyped mannerisms is *catatonia*. It was first described as a consequence of intense emotional anguish and tension.[1] Although it frequently responds to sedative drugs, electroshock is the more complete and effective treatment.

Catatonia is a feature of several mental disorders; it can appear suddenly and immobilize the patient. When it is transient it can be disregarded, but when it persists it can dominate the mental state and behavior and threaten the patient's life if he fails to eat. Catatonia takes a terrible toll in forced feedings, bedsores resulting from immobility, muscular atrophy, bladder catheterizations and consequent infection, and blood clots in immobilized limbs. If the clots move to the lungs or brain they can cause death or stroke.[2]

The condition is seen in patients with affective illnesses—both depression and mania—in patients with systemic disorders, and in those with toxic brain states caused by hallucinogenic drugs.[3] For decades the prevailing belief in psychiatry was that each instance of catatonia represented a subtype of schizophrenia. The major classification systems in psychiatry—DSM-III of the American Psychiatric Association (1980, 1987) and the International Classification of Diseases (ICD-IX, ICD-X)—assigned to all patients with catatonia the diagnosis of schizophrenia, catatonic type. As a consequence, few of these patients were treated with sedatives or with electroshock, because those treatments are not recommended for schizophrenia.[4] This error was rectified to a small extent in the 1994 classification system of the American Psychiatric Association (DSM-IV), which recognized a form of catatonia as a feature of mood disorders.[5]

The presence of catatonia is defined by two or more characteristic motor signs in a patient with a mental disorder.[6] There are many types of catatonia, including an acute form with high risk for death, labeled *pernicious catatonia* or *malignant catatonia*. The *neuroleptic malignant syndrome*, which may follow the administration of neuroleptic drugs, is a special instance.[7]

Catatonia may be transitory or may, if untreated, persist for months or years. It responds to the intravenous administration of barbiturates or benzodiazepines. The barbiturate Amytal was the usual intervention until the merits of the benzodiazepines Ativan and Valium were recognized. When these medications fail, as they do in about 10 percent of the cases, the syndrome can be effectively and quickly relieved by ECT, which cures the syndrome, in almost all cases, within three treatments.

GERALD LEE, a 20-year-old college student who had been studying intensively for end-of-semester tests and getting little sleep, was found by his parents sitting like stone in front of the television screen. For days he refused to answer questions and did not sleep, eat, or bathe. When his parents brought him to the psychiatric emergency room, he stayed seated, rigid, silent, and staring into space. An intravenous injection of Ativan soon relieved the motor aspects of the illness, and Gerald then told of voices instructing him not to speak, of messages personally directed at him from the television set, and of his fears that he would soon die. Within an hour he was again mute, staring, and oblivious of his surroundings.

No evidence of toxic drugs was found in his urine and blood, but only repeated intravenous injections of Ativan enabled him to feed himself and use the toilet. After a physical examination and laboratory tests showed no systemic cause for his behavior, he was described as having acute schizophrenia of the catatonia type. The use of antipsychotic drugs was rejected because of the possibility that they could bring about neuroleptic malignant syndrome, which is possible in a patient with signs of catatonia. At that point, the risks and benefits of ECT were discussed with Mr. Lee's parents, who gave consent for the treatments.

Immediately after the third treatment of bilateral ECT, Mr. Lee was responsive, pleasant, cooperative, and bewildered by the descriptions of his recent behavior. He recalled hearing voices but could not explain their origin. He asked to be allowed to return to school, and, though continuation ECT was recommended, he refused, insisting that he was well. He did agree to continue taking lithium.

After two weeks in school, he was brought back to the hospital, staring, rigid, and posturing. Ativan again erased the immediate syndrome, but even high doses did not sustain the effect. Electroshock again brought relief, after just five treatments. This time, Mr. Lee agreed to continuation ECT. He received four treatments weekly and then six additional biweekly treatments while he attended a daytime hospital program. He also took lithium and Ativan and, after four months, returned to school, where he kept up his regular classwork.

Almost a year later, however, his parents brought him back to the hospital with the same syndrome, which was relieved this time by a course of 11 ECT. Because a urine examination showed signs of kidney dysfunction, Tegretol was prescribed in place of lithium. Mr. Lee decided not to complete his schooling; he took a job in a manufacturing assembly plant and has remained well for more than two years.

Comment. Mr. Lee's immediate response to ECT was misinterpreted as recovery, and he was justified in refusing continuation treatment. Since the benefits of ECT, like those of psychotropic medicines, are transient, patients require repeated and extensive treatment for a sustained effect.

Neuroleptic malignant syndrome (NMS)

Fever, motor rigidity, negativism, mutism, and heart and respiratory instability are components of *neuroleptic malignant syndrome*, which may appear after the administration of antipsychotic drugs. The syndrome is indistinguishable from catatonia, except that a specific precipitant has been identified, usually one of the high-potency neuroleptic drugs like Haldol, Prolixin, or Navane. Cases have been observed in association with almost all neuroleptics, including the recently introduced "atypical" Clozaril and Risperdol. This syndrome is sometimes responsive to the simple remedies of supportive fluids and rest, and withdrawal of the offending substances. When those fail to help, though, electroshock is usually successful.

Whether NMS is a specific consequence of an excessive reduction in the amount of brain dopamine or whether it is a type of catatonia is still undetermined.[8] Those who see it as a specific disorder in dopamine activity seek to increase brain dopamine by prescribing Parlodel or Sinemet and to relieve muscular rigidity and fever through the use of the muscle relaxant Dentrium.[9] Neither of these treatments is specifically effective. ECT is the definitive and effective treatment for NMS.[10]

JEFFREY COOPER, a 40-year-old, had been treated for schizophrenia with antipsychotic and antimanic medications since he was 16. He was stabilized on Thorazine and lithium therapy and had been attending a community clinic for the prescription of his psychotropic medicines. His therapist, encouraged by the persisting relief of his symptoms, decided to reduce his doses, then switched him to the new atypical neuroleptic Zyprexa. One month later, Mr. Cooper again became psychotic, and the traditional neuroleptic Trilafon was prescribed. He quickly became febrile, mute, and rigid; the diagnosis of NMS was made, and he was transferred to a tertiary care hospital.

The neuroleptic drugs were discontinued and Mr. Cooper was treated with large doses of Parlodel and Dentrium. His repetitive motor movements prompted the diagnosis of epilepsy, so anticonvulsants were administered. Ativan, in low doses, controlled his infrequent agitation. He remained mute and rigid and required total nursing care. A permanent opening to his stomach from his abdomen, a gastrostomy, was done to permit feeding. Because he was immobilized, he developed pulmonary and bladder infections, which required the use of antibiotics.

A visiting lecturer and consultant happened to see the patient after Mr. Cooper had been in intensive medical care for four months. The consultant agreed with the diagnosis of catatonia but recommended Ativan at doses higher than had been used. When the doses were increased to 12 mg/day, Mr. Cooper, for the first time in months, responded to commands and smiled at his parents, though he remained mute.

ECT was recommended by the visiting lecturer, who continued to consult on the case, but it was not available at the tertiary care center so Mr. Cooper was transferred to another academic center. When his mother was signing the consent form for ECT, she recalled that her son had had a similar episode of psychosis, rigidity, and mutism when he was 16 and he had responded well to ECT.

The Ativan was reduced to 6 mg/day, and bilateral ECT was administered every other day. After the fifth treatment, he was alert, responsive, and friendly; he recognized his parents, tried to talk, smiled, was less rigid, and took oral feedings. By the ninth treatment he was verbally responsive to his parents and the professional staff. The four months of rigidity and forced bed rest, however, had left him with limb strictures and such badly impaired movement that he was unable to stand or to use his hands to feed himself.

The Ativan was increased to 8 mg/day, and ECT sessions were spaced at weekly intervals. As the patient became more verbal he expressed psychotic thoughts, and the treatment team had to decide whether to administer neuroleptics or increase the frequency of ECT. A single 2.5 mg dose of Moban resulted in an immediate autonomic crisis with elevated serum creatinine phosphokinase (CPK), signs of an incipient NMS, so it was discontinued. A few days later, Zyprexa was added to ECT at 10-day intervals and Ativan at 7 mg/day. Immediately after each treatment, catatonia and psychosis were less prominent, but they recurred over three to five days. Since the Zyprexa seemed of little benefit, Clozaril was started.

At this juncture, Mr. Cooper was no longer psychotic and no longer exhibited signs of catatonia. He could use both of his hands, with some residual restriction in movement, and he was able to stand. After 22 treatments, he was transferred to a rehabilitation center, where he was actively interested in his progress and began to use his hands to feed himself. The prognosis for recovery was good.

Comment. Jeffrey Cooper's case is an example of persistent catatonia and inadequate treatment. The failure to consider adequate doses of benzodiazepines and ECT stemmed from the mistaken belief that NMS is a specific entity, separate from catatonia, with a different treatment algorithm.

Because the tertiary care center to which Mr. Cooper was sent did not have the resources for administering ECT, he was transferred once again. At the first center, the staff had not considered ECT for Jeffrey because it was not within their experience. That a tertiary care hospital, licensed to treat mentally ill patients could not itself provide ECT is an unhappy comment on the lack of understanding of the treatment's merits.

Another syndrome, the toxic serotonin syndrome, has recently been recognized as a response to some of the newer antidepressant drugs, known as *selective serotonin reuptake inhibitors* (SSRI). Prozac, Zoloft, and Paxil are the best-known medicines of this class, and the syndrome has been reported with each. The motor and mental changes are similar to those of NMS. While the role of electroshock in treating the syndrome has yet to be defined, it is expected to be of benefit when the more practical remedies of supportive fluids, rest, and withdrawal of the offending substances do not help.[11]

Parkinsonism

Many depressed patients, especially the elderly, are slow and hesitant in movement, rigid in posture, and tremulous. When they are treated for depression with electroshock, both the motor signs and the depressed mood are relieved.[12] This motor syndrome is hardly distinguishable from Parkinson's disease caused by cerebrovascular change or systemic infection. To separate the effects of ECT on parkinsonism from its effects on depression, Swedish scientists studied hospitalized patients suffering from a severe form of parkinsonism who were not depressed. Using real and sham ECT, they found that real ECT relieved the rigidity of parkinsonism but not the tremor.[13] These observations have been confirmed, and ECT is an accepted treatment for parkinsonism marked by severe rigidity, independent of the presence of a mood disorder.[14]

ROBERT MONROE, 72 years old, developed bilateral parkinsonism when he was 63. Treatment with anti-Parkinson agents was successful for about seven years, but after that the medications gave him only a few hours of relief from severe stiffness and moderate tremor. He spent his time mainly in bed or in a chair and needed assistance in feeding and going to the toilet. Though he was depressed, he did not express thoughts of self-harm or develop psychosis or melancholia. Although he received some help from the anti-Parkinson regimens of Sinemet and anticholinergic agents Cogentin and Artane, Mr. Monroe was unhappy about the limitations on his activities. He was alert and well-oriented, even though he could not stand or walk unaided and could speak only slowly in a hoarse, uncertain voice. A review and examination found no signs of other systemic illness.

When he and his wife were told of an experimental protocol approved by a university for a trial of electroshock in patients with parkinsonism, they gave their consent. He continued his anti-Parkinson medications at the full dosage.

Immediately after the third bilateral ECT, Mr. Monroe spent a full day out of bed. He was able to feed and tend to himself and to speak more clearly. That night, however, he had nightmares, and the next day he was delirious, frightened, and unable to say where he was. His heart rate was rapid and blood pressure elevated. Sinemet was discontinued, and the syndrome abated. Three days later he was once again well-oriented though stiff.

The delirium he experienced was ascribed to dopamine toxicity occasioned by the combination of continued Sinemet (which is changed in the body to brain dopamine) and the brain dopamine released by ECT. One week after the dose of Sinemet was reduced by half, ECT was reinstated. His motor rigidity eased. After three ECT he was able to walk with assistance and to leave his bed at will. The mental disturbances did not recur.

After 11 treatments, given twice a week, Mr. Monroe went

home and continued outpatient ECT at alternating weekly and biweekly sessions for four months. Throughout the course of treatment, except for the period of acute toxicity, he remained oriented. He did occasionally complain of forgetfulness. An avid card player, he continued to play gin rummy (and win as before). With the arrival of winter, he moved to Florida, where his outpatient care was maintained, the treatments given less frequently until, after 10 months, they were stopped. His Parkinson's symptoms were relieved with lower doses of Sinemet, and he continued his homebound life with tolerable rigidity and tremor.

Comment. Repeated seizures stimulate the tissues to liberate increased amounts of brain neurohumors. Dopamine is the brain neurohumor that is deficient in patients with parkinsonism, caused by aging, vascular or infectious disease, or prolonged use of neuroleptic drugs. ECT relieves the rigidity occasioned by each of these causes. The application of electroshock in treating parkinsonism is still considered experimental, but it is being called on with increasing frequency.

Now that the risks of delirium from full-dosage anti-Parkinson agents are recognized, these medications are reduced before ECT is begun.[15]

Toxic syndromes

The hallucinogenic drugs cocaine, amphetamine, lysergide (LSD), and cannabis (marijuana) often elicit states of excitement with paranoid ideation. Such states are responsive to electroshock.

ERIC NEWTON, a 15-year-old, was referred to the hospital when he became irritable, had inappropriate verbal outbursts, and showed unprovoked aggressive behavior, slept and ate excessively, and put on 10 pounds in a few weeks. He had been sleepless for two days, and said that he was being watched by neighbors. At times, instead of overeating, he refused food and remained alone in his room.

Following an intravenous injection of Amytal, Eric talked of having smoked cannabis during the weekend. He was preoccupied with thoughts of death, and his threat of suicide necessitated continuous nursing protection. At times he became so distressed that he required physical restraint.

A similar episode had occurred five months earlier, when he was a patient in a community hospital and experienced a single grand mal seizure, followed by belligerency, aggressivity, and hypersexuality. The urine examination at that time was positive for cannabinoids. He was treated with antipsychotic drugs, but even with low doses he became rigid, mute, sedated, and febrile. When the medications were withheld, he recovered and returned to school after three weeks.

At this earlier hospital admission, ECT was recommended, and, with parental consent, he received three treatments in four days. By the second treatment, the depressed mood and delusional thoughts disappeared, and he spoke spontaneously. After the third treatment, he was bright, cheerful, friendly, and pleasant, with a good appetite and normal sleep rhythms. Following an additional nine days without relapse, he was discharged to home and school.

Eric continued in psychotherapy. He told his therapist that each time he smoked marijuana he became ill, so he had not used it since his last hospitalization. He performed well in high school, graduating in the upper quarter of his class. Four years later he is married, working, and the father of a child.

Comment. Eric Newton suffered from a cannabis-induced psychosis with suicidal and catatonic features. He did not tolerate neuroleptics. The efficacy of ECT in relieving his manic features reflects its safety and efficacy. Similar success of ECT is reported in treating toxic delusional states caused by LSD and PCP.[16]

Self-injury

Repetitive compulsive acts mark a number of abnormal mental states—the hand-washing by patients with obsessive-compulsive disorder, the symbolic slashing of wrists in patients with borderline personality disorder, and the repetitive face-scratching and head-banging of patients with mental retardation. These movement syndromes are occasionally responsive to electroshock.

DONALD PAINE, a 14-year-old retarded boy, was admitted to a university inpatient facility because of his persistent headbanging, which required him to wear a protective helmet and be restrained most of the day. His mental age was defined as 4.3

years. Donald's communication was mainly by interpretable gut-
tural sounds. The head-banging and skin-scratching began when
he was 10 and persisted despite extensive medication and both
positive and negative reinforcement. He wore large gloves in addition to the helmet, and was sedated to control his high-pitched
wailing and prolonged screaming. After four years of failed treatment, a consultant suggested evaluation for a trial of ECT, which
is when we saw him.

Donald was receiving Tegretol, lithium, and Navane, and a systemic examination found no disorders to preclude further treatment. Considering the long list of treatments that had been tried
without success, a course of ECT seemed reasonable. Consent was
obtained from his legal guardian, lithium was discontinued, and
Tegretol and Navane were continued.

After the sixth treatment of twice-weekly bilateral ECT, Donald's screaming, scratching, and head-banging were reduced. By
the tenth treatment, he no longer needed the helmet and gloves
or the restraints. Treatments were reduced to once weekly, and
after 16 treatments he was returned to his residence. For an additional two months, treatments were given once every two weeks
and then stopped, because the psychiatrists were satisfied with the
progress. Anticonvulsants and the atypical neuroleptic Risperdal
were prescribed, and no life-threatening behavior has been evident
for two years.

Comment. The decrease in head-banging in this retarded young
man is consistent with the improvement effected by ECT in other
repetitive acts. Obsessive thoughts and compulsive acts, the hand-
wringing of agitated depression, the stereotyped motor acts of catatonia, and the self-inflicted injuries of the mentally retarded also
improve with ECT. However, in the past these good responses
were usually short-lived. It seems likely that the relapses occurred
because of the short courses of ECT that were common before the
1990s. Continuation ECT is now more readily available and, if the
courses are adequate, is frequently beneficial. In Donald's case, the
treatments were spread over four months, a period known to be
effective in patients with such severe conditions.

Donald's court-appointed legal guardian only reluctantly, and
after much persuasion, allowed ECT to be administered. In stating
his belief that electroshock was dangerous and abusive to his cli-

ent, he was reflecting the common confusion about ECT and the use of high-energy electric shocks to condition behavior in an animal or a human. In fact, electric shocks—delivered with devices known as cattle prods—to teach a child or animal that certain acts will be painful was once a conditioning therapy used among the mentally retarded. Those experiments, rightly condemned, are no longer in use. But apprehension about the abuse of the mentally ill with electricity was so broadly circulated that it is still difficult for doctors to apply the treatment. The public misinformation is tragic; it can deprive mentally ill patients of a useful treatment.

Intractable seizure disorders

Seizure disorders occasionally become intractable and persist as uncontrollable fits, known as status epilepticus (SE). SE is an emergency condition that is associated with high morbidity and a mortality rate of 20 percent in adults.[17] Treatment is difficult, usually calling for rapidly increased doses of anticonvulsant medications and, eventually, general anesthesia.[18]

During a course of convulsive therapy, the brain's seizure threshold rises, and it becomes more difficult to elicit a seizure. In 1943, Kalinowsky and Kennedy demonstrated the feasibility of curtailing SE by superimposing electroshock seizures. Their observation has been repeatedly confirmed.[19]

The pathophysiology of SE is the persistence of a low seizure threshold, despite repeated seizures, with a failure of the biochemical inhibitory mechanisms to rise to levels that are sufficient to terminate a seizure. In SE the seizures, although frequent, are not robust, as found in studies of prolactin in the blood serum. In a robust seizure, like that developed during ECT and like many epileptic seizures, the concentration of prolactin in the blood increases markedly.[20] The measurement of serum prolactin in the hour after a seizure differentiates true epileptic seizures from hysterical or pseudo-seizures.[21] In SE, prolactin levels do not rise; indeed, they remain normal both in adults and in children.[22] This failure of patients in SE to release large amounts of prolactin suggests that their seizures are incomplete and cannot stimulate a robust inhibitory termination process. But maximal seizures can be elicited with ECT even in SE, which makes ECT a reasonable alternative to general anesthesia.[23]

Chapter 9

How Does It Work?

The major puzzle about ECT is how it works. How do seizures, which can be dangerous and damaging when they occur spontaneously, become beneficial? Ladislas Meduna, the originator of convulsive therapy, believed in a biological antagonism between psychosis and seizures, an antagonism we no longer consider credible. But though we may smile at the belief, we acknowledge that it led him to devise methods to induce seizures safely, select the patient who was likely to benefit, develop a protocol for a successful course of treatments, demonstrate the safety of induced seizures, evaluate the merits and risks of treatment, and convince others to continue his work. His observations have been repeatedly verified, leaving little doubt as to the effectiveness of convulsive therapy in treating mental illnesses.

We know a great deal about the essentials of a successful course of ECT.[1] Neither anesthesia nor electric current alone is useful, nor, except rarely, is a single seizure.[2] To be of benefit, seizures must be repeated two or three times a week for many weeks. The more recent the mood, thought, or movement disorder, the more fully it can be relieved. Cases involving lifelong problems, character pathology, neuroses, and the mood disorders secondary to the abuse of drugs are not amenable to treatment. We know how to avoid the risks of anoxia, unmodified convulsions, and prolonged seizures, and to recognize that these aspects of the treatment course do not explain how ECT works.

The neuroendocrine system

Endocrine glands play dominant roles in our lives. The products of the glands control life's cycles, from daily feeding and sleeping, growth and maturation, sex and fetal development, to senescence and death. In contrast to the brain's neurohumors, which act briefly and locally at the points of contacts (synapses) between neurons, hormones are discharged into the bloodstream to be distributed to all the cells of the body. The principal glands are the thyroid and parathyroid in the neck, the adrenal glands above the kidneys, specialized cells in the pancreas, and the sex glands of the ovary and testes. The main controlling glands are the hypothalamus and the pituitary at the base of the brain. The substances of one gland affect the release and activity of the others. They operate in an interacting rheostatic system, with hormones normally released in daily rhythms, as pulsatile discharges, rising with wakefulness and falling with sleep.[3]

An example is the release of cortisol, the adrenal hormone that is controlled by the adrenocorticotrophic hormone (ACTH) of the pituitary gland.[4] The release of cortisol, in turn, inhibits the release of ACTH. The amount of cortisol in the blood and in the urine changes with the sleep-wake cycle—highest when we are awake and lowest just as we fall asleep. The traveler who crosses time zones knows what hormone disruption can do to the body. Because his sleep cycle and the cyclic release of cortisol are disrupted, he experiences changes in mood and wakefulness, fatigue, loss of concentration, impaired memory, and dulled mood. Once the traveler adjusts to the new time cycle, the cortisol release cycle is re-established, and those symptoms disappear.

The effects of any endocrine gland dysfunction can be equally widespread. If the thyroid fails to produce enough of its hormones, the result is hypothyroidism. If that defect occurs in early childhood, the outcome is extreme mental deficiency. If it occurs in an adult, the syndrome is known as myxedema. Fluids accumulate in the person's body tissues, his mental activity lags, his muscles become weak, and his reflexes and the electrical rhythms of his brain become very slow. He is depressed and has poor memory and paranoid thoughts. Coma, even death, may follow. On the other hand, if the thyroid gland secretes excessive amounts of hormones, his behavior is marked by excitement, mania, and grandiosity. Similar systemic and mental effects have been associated with deficiencies or excesses of the hormones produced by the pituitary, hypothalamus, adrenal, parathyroid, testis, and ovary glands.

A neuroendocrine view of ECT

One of the remarkable findings of modern psychiatric research is that the hormones in patients with mental illnesses are wildly disordered. The pair of adrenal glands in a depressed person produce too much cortisol, the high levels in the blood disrupt the normal diurnal rhythm, and the glands fail to respond to the usual feedback mechanisms. The most prominent features of depression—failure to eat, loss of weight, inability to sleep, loss of interest in sex, inability to concentrate thoughts, and difficulties in memory—dominate the body, because these functions are intimately regulated by the pituitary and the adrenal glands acting in tandem.

Each seizure stimulates the hypothalamus to discharge its hormones. Those stimulate the pituitary gland to discharge its products, which then inhibit the discharge of cortisol from the adrenal glands. The first effects are transitory, but by the fourth or fifth seizure, the normal interaction of the hormones of the hypothalamic-pituitary-adrenal axis is again in place. Feeding and sleep become normal; then motor activity, mood, memory, and thought follow suit.

How does a seizure cause such profound changes in physiology? Although epileptic fits may arise from any portion of the brain, only those that come from the central part of the brain—the brain stem or centrencephalic structures—are essential to electroshock's favorable effects. The hormonal cells of the hypothalamus sit right above, and are intimately related to, the cells of the pituitary gland. In electroshock, the currents from the stimulating electrodes on each temple pass through the central parts of the brain, and stimulate both the hypothalamus to discharge its hormones and the centrencephalic structures to express a bilateral grand mal seizure.[5] The lesser efficacy of unilateral electrode placement, in fact, results from the currents having to take indirect routes in order to affect these areas of the brain.[6]

Mental disorders arise when specialized brain cells lack the materials they need to function properly. During ECT, large amounts of hypothalamic and pituitary hormones are "squeezed out" and new levels are measurable in the cerebrospinal fluid (CSF) and the blood within a few minutes.[7]

The brain's structure helps us understand how the chemicals

released by seizures are made available to brain cells. The brain consists of two large hemispheres that sit atop a central brain stem. These hemispheres are not solid structures like the liver or spleen, but are hollow. The sac-like structures, known as the lateral ventricles, are fluid-filled spaces that are connected to another sac (third ventricle), which lines the space between the two hemispheres. Behind these, and connected to them, is a fourth ventricle, sitting above the brain stem and below the cerebellum. The fluid-filled ventricles are also connected to the spaces on the surfaces of the brain and the full length of the spinal cord. By these intricate sacs and pathways, all the brain's cells are bathed by a clear, watery cerebrospinal fluid containing many chemical substances identified as peptides, amino acids, neurohumors, and proteins. These chemicals come from brain cells and from the body's endocrine glands via the blood stream. The fluid is produced continuously in the brain and circulation is assured by highly vascular structures (chorioid plexus) in the ventricles that absorb CSF and pass it to the blood.

Richard Bergland (1985), a neurosurgeon, asked what the role of the CSF and the brain's ventricular system may play in the brain's physiology.[8] Using paper chromatography, a method that separates substances dissolved in a fluid, he observed more than 300 different peptides and amino acids in the CSF. He induced seizures in sheep, extracted CSF from the ventricles, and found the substances to substantially increase in variety and in amount after seizures.

The brain's ventricular system makes the substances carried in the CSF accessible to all brain cells, which extract what they need to properly function. Picture the CSF as a conveyer belt, allowing brain cells to pick up this peptide now, another later, and more of yet another as the cell demands. That is what you and I do when we go to a food buffet; we select what we need now, and pass up others. At another time our selections differ, as our needs differ. It is not so strange that electroshock corrects so many different disorders, since it unselectively increases the availability of many different substances that are needed for different specialized functions.

An example of this process is seen in the relief of parkinsonism. Motor rigidity, tremors, and hesitant gait result when the brain's substantia nigra lacks dopamine, a neurohumor. Physicians prescribe large doses of *l*-dopa, a precursor of dopamine, to encourage the brain to produce more dopamine. When the prescription is successful, brain dopamine levels increase, the rigidity that inhibited proper easy movement decreases, and body movements become smooth again. When *l*-dopa treatment fails, electroshock is used; it also floods the CSF with dopamine, relieving parkinsonian patients of rigidity and hesitant gait.

For many patients, the effects of a small series of treatments persist for long periods after the course ends. At other times, the brain cells again function poorly and the mental disorder re-emerges. In such cases, ECT is continued to sustain normal brain cellular functions and a normal mental state.

We assume that brain cells regulate mood, thought, memory, and motor functions by different hormones.[9] Admittedly, we have not yet identified specific substances with effects on mood and thought analogous to insulin's effect on sugar metabolism, thyroxin's effect on cellular metabolism, and parathormone's effect on calcium metabolism. The lack of identification of behavior-regulating substances is often cited as criticism of the neuro-endocrine view of the mode of action of electroshock, but the criticism cannot negate the empirical evidence that such substances exist.[10] It is reasonable that ventricular fluids be examined before and after seizures to find substances that either appear anew or are changed in amount. The identification of such substances will mark those that we may ethically search for in patients. Such a search should make possible the development of an effective replacement for ECT.[11]

Chapter 10

∞

The Origins of Electroshock Therapy

Modern psychiatry began in the latter half of the 19th century with the identification, by European neuropsychiatrists, of separate mental disorders. At the time, three mental illnesses dominated the clinical scene: neurosyphilis, described as dementia paralytica, dementia praecox (schizophrenia today), and manic-depressive insanity (major depression and bipolar disorder today).

At the beginning of the 20th century, no effective treatments were known. Caretakers of the mentally ill commonly resorted to chains, restraining chairs, cold and hot baths, and seclusion. Morphine, bromides, barbiturates, and chloral hydrate kept patients asleep but did little to heal their illnesses. The mentally ill who were dangerous to themselves or to others were housed in large state-supported hospitals, managed by hospital superintendents with full authority to treat the inmates. Lacking effective treatments, they permitted many "experimental" and unsafe interventions.

Agitated patients were subjected to prolonged sleep and stupefaction for days.[1] The few who seemed to recover their senses—many died of pneumonia—encouraged doctors to continue such trials. Bodily infection was considered a cause of mental disorder, so teeth, tonsils, gall bladder, and large sections of the colon were removed, even though there was no experimental evidence to justify the procedures. Many patients died. Those who survived suffered further humiliation because the hospitals did not provide false teeth to help the patients chew their food.[2]

Surgical removal of sexual organs—salpingectomy (closure of the Fallopian tubes in women) and vasectomy (tying the vas deferens in men)—was another "treatment." The eugenics movement was active in the United States in response to large waves of immigrants, and eugenicists argued for sterilization of those with mental illness.[3] In 1907, state lawmakers in Indiana made mandatory the sterilization of criminals, idiots, imbeciles, and rapists. By 1940, 30 states had such laws, and it is estimated that more than 18,000 people in psychiatric institutions were surgically sterilized during those years.[4]

The discovery of bacterial pathogens as the cause of infectious febrile illnesses was a great accomplishment of medical research in the 19th century. Pasteur's demonstration that high temperatures would destroy bacteria, an observation that led to the pasteurization of foods, suggested that fevers could have a therapeutic benefit. Occasional reports of improvement of psychosis in patients who had smallpox or typhoid fever suggested that fever could also ameliorate mental disorders, but because high fevers could be lethal, ways were sought to control them.[5]

Syphilis, a sexually transmitted disease that is often fatal, affects all body tissues. No effective treatment was known, and patients were subjected to large doses of arsenic and mercury, systemic poisons comparable to the chemotherapy prescribed for cancer patients today. The most devastating form of the disease, neurosyphilis, the infection of the brain and spinal cord by a spirochete, manifests itself years after the causative sexual exposure. It was as widespread and as feared a disease as HIV and AIDS are today. Neurosyphilis mimics the symptoms of every mental disorder: personality change, dementia, delirium, paranoia, depression, mania, and muscular paralysis. It slowly and relentlessly and painfully leads to death.

In its chronic and progressive form, syphilis does not stimulate fever, the body's defense, so scientists sought ways to bring it about. The discovery that quinine could effectively treat malaria, a disease with recurrent high fevers, made it possible for Professor Wagner-Jauregg, of the University of Vienna, to test the effects of fever on neurosyphilis. In 1917, he transfused the blood of a malarial seaman into nine neurosyphilitic patients, each of whom developed malaria with high fever in 48-to 96-hour cycles. After six to 10 episodes, usually within three to four weeks, the infections were cleared by large doses of quinine. Three of the patients recovered, three were much improved, and three were unchanged by the treatment. None died. Wagner-Jauregg's report was published in 1918, and his work brought him the Nobel Prize in Medicine in 1927.[6]

Success in controlling neurosyphilis by malarial fever therapy varied from 8 percent to 51 percent. Attempts to induce fevers by other means were not much better.[7] There was little agreement as to how many fevers should be induced, or for what length of time they were to be maintained. Some authors, including Wagner-Jauregg, accepted eight to 10 malarial fevers as effective; others, embarrassed by their low success rates, encouraged up to 50 daily fevers.

Fever therapy's complications—dehydration, circulatory collapse, cerebral anoxia, and surgical shock—led to death rates reported from different hospitals of 2 percent to 47 percent. Yet, despite the low success rate and high incidence of complications and death, so feared was neurosyphilis as a mental illness and as a fatal disease that fever therapy was internationally accepted until it was replaced by penicillin in 1944.[8]

This "success" of malarial fever in treating neurosyphilis led to a widely discussed theory of the antagonism of diseases used as medicine, relying on the introduction of one disease to cure another. This idea was the basis for using convulsive therapy as a treatment for dementia praecox, another devastating mental disease.

Chemical convulsive therapy

Patients with dementia praecox who developed epileptic seizures after a head injury or after encephalitis were occasionally cured of their mental disorder. Because the pattern suggested a biological antagonism between dementia praecox and epilepsy, some physicians sought to halt intractable epilepsy with transfusions of the blood of psychotic patients, hoping that a chemical product of the psychosis in the blood would counteract and treat epilepsy. The efforts failed.[9]

In the early 1930s, Ladislas Meduna, a physician trained in neurology and neuropathology, was examining human postmortem specimens at the Hungarian Psychiatric Research Institute in Budapest.[10] Meduna observed that the brains of patients with dementia praecox had fewer than the normal number of neuroglia and that the brains of patients with epilepsy had markedly more. The neuroglia are the myriads of branched cells in the central nervous system that provide a supporting and communicating network for the neurons, the main cells of the brain that are the basis for thought, memory, emotion, and action. Meduna theorized that the deficiency was a sign of dementia praecox and inferred that the amelioration of the symptoms of dementia praecox in patients who developed epileptic seizures must be due to the increase in the number of neuroglia.[11]

Could artificial seizures increase those cells? He examined various substances for their seizure-inducing potential in animals and settled on the intramuscular injection of camphor-in-oil.[12] After 15 to 60 minutes it produced a grand mal convulsion that did not incapacitate or kill the animal. The technique seemed applicable to humans.

But many clinicians, including the director of the Hungarian Psychiatric Institute, believed that dementia praecox was an inherited genetic disorder and was therefore irremediable. The idea that dementia praecox might be treatable was academic heresy. Fearing criticism, Meduna moved his research activities from the institute to a state hospital for the long-term mentally ill at Lipotmezö, outside Budapest.

Among his patients was Zoltan, a 33-year-old man who had been psychotic, mute, and withdrawn for four years. Zoltan, who required feeding through a tube, suffered from dementia praecox of the catatonic type, and, since all other measures had failed, was deemed suitable for experimental treatment.

On January 23, 1934, Meduna injected camphor-in-oil into an arm muscle, and "after 45 minutes of anxious and fearful waiting the patient suddenly had a classical epileptic attack that lasted 60 seconds." Zoltan recovered from the seizure without harm.[13]

Following the model of malarial treatment for neurosyphilis, Meduna repeated the injections at three-to four-day intervals.

Two days after the fifth injection, on February 10 in the morning, for the first time in four years, he got out of his bed, began to talk, requested breakfast, dressed himself without help, was interested in everything around him, and asked about his disease and how long he had been in the hospital. When we told him he spent 4 years at the hospital, he did not believe it.

Injections were repeated three more times, and Zoltan's symptoms were sufficiently relieved that he returned home. He was well when Meduna left Europe in 1939.

Meduna treated five other patients with camphor, and each of them improved. Learning that intravenous injections of Metrazol had safely induced seizures in animals, Meduna tried this compound in place of camphor. He found Metrazol easier to use, and because the seizures it induced were immediate and predictable, Metrazol quickly became the principal agent. During the next two years, Meduna treated 110 patients, and in 1937 he reported relief and remission of mental illness in 53 of them.[14] Among those who had been ill for less than four years, the remission rate was higher. The seizures elicited by Metrazol and those elicited by camphor were equally effective, suggesting that the therapy was inherent in the seizure, not in the mode of induction. That conclusion led directly to seizures elicited by electricity.

Within six months of the publication of an interim report in 1935, Meduna received visitors from Italy, Germany, India, Australia, and the United States. In May 1937, he discussed the Metrazol treatment at an international meeting organized by the Swiss Neuropsychiatric Society.[15] He was then invited to lecture throughout Europe, South America, and the United States. While he was on an invited lecture tour to South America, Meduna heard of the invasion of Austria-Hungary by the Nazis, and he sought asylum in the United States. He worked in Chicago until his death in 1964.[16]

Electroconvulsive therapy

The induction of a seizure by Metrazol was a frightening procedure. Within a few minutes after the intravenous injection, the patient's thoughts began to race, his heart beat more rapidly, he experienced feelings of terror and impending doom—and suddenly lost consciousness.[17] When he awakened, his muscles and back ached, often his tongue and lips were bleeding, and he had a violent headache. Many patients refused further treatment. Making the procedure less unpleasant was imperative. Electric currents were tested in many animal experiments, and a successful method was designed.[18]

A 39-year-old man, suffering from a manic and psychotic episode, was admitted to the University Hospital in Rome. He had had a similar episode a few years earlier, at which time he had responded well to Metrazol therapy. Now, on April 11, 1938, he became the first person in whom a seizure was induced electrically.

A team headed by Ugo Cerletti and Luigi Bini initially applied a current that was subconvulsive. A second induction, at a higher setting, immediately induced a grand mal seizure. Seizures were repeated on alternate days over the next three weeks, and the patient recovered.[19]

Metrazol convulsive treatments had already galvanized psychiatric practice; the use of electricity in its stead stimulated further interest.[20] When physicians emigrated from Italy to England and the United States, they brought with them the instruments they had used, or they had instruments built in their new locations according to the original designs.[21] By 1940 electroshock therapy was as widely used as Metrazol convulsive therapy.

Other drastic interventions

At the same time that the chemical and electrical convulsive therapies were developed, the profession learned of two other interventions to relieve schizophrenia: insulin coma, introduced by Manfred Sakel in Vienna in 1933, and lobotomy, the ablation of the frontal lobes of the brain, developed by Egas Moniz in Lisbon in 1935. The three forms of treatment, which all became known within a brief span, were intimately related in the minds of the public and the profession. When neither insulin coma nor lobotomy was found to be effective, each was supplanted by the psychotropic drugs introduced in the 1950s. By the time ECT was once again called on (in the 1970s) to treat medication-resistant cases, its image had been tarnished by the almost universal confusion of this method with the two abandoned interventions.

As with the desperate interventions developed for neurosyphilis and schizophrenia, chance, adventurism, bravado, and disregard for scientific investigation set off a rash of treatments that were most often applied without formal testing for efficacy or for safety. The medical literature contains claims for many untested means of dealing with the psychoneuroses and psychoses. Other unproven therapies for the psychoses included sleep deprivation, continuous sleep, acetylcholine infusions, nitrous oxide, ether inhalation, histamine injections, megavitamins and complex diets, atropine and scopolamine coma, hemodialysis, intravenous lysergide (LSD), methamphetamine and megimide, hypothermia, photoshock, regressive electroshock, subcoma insulin, cerebral pneumotherapy, high-dose reserpine, acupuncture, and light therapy.

Similarly heroic treatments were considered for psychoneuroses, those disorders identified as hysterical amnesia, phobia, obsessive-compulsive disorder, and hypochondriasis. Among the unproven psychotherapies are psychoanalysis, its various modifications for individual therapy, group therapy, family therapy, milieu and psychosocial therapies, behavior therapy, client-centered psychotherapy, cognitive therapy, hypnotherapy, existential and marital therapy. Several are actively practiced today.

The audacity of Wagner-Jauregg, Meduna, Cerletti, and Bini, and the many others who sought to alter the course of mental illness by physical means, was abetted by the patients' view of their doctors as paternalistic figures.[22] It was assumed that doctors' efforts were always for the benefit of their patients. The doctors' boldness, in turn, was encouraged by the hopeless nature of many mental disorders as well as the willingness of patients to endure any hardship, suffer any risk, and pay any price for relief.[23] But many were treated unwillingly, and even despite their protests. Once a patient was admitted to a psychiatric facility, his consent was assumed and his refusal was given no heed. Such incidents led to public dismay and anger, which spurred legislative attempts to interdict psychiatric treatments and limit their use to voluntary, mentally competent patients who could and did consent. The concept of voluntary consent for somatic treatment of the mentally ill was initially shaped by the consent procedure for electroshock drawn up by a task force of the American Psychiatric Association in 1978.[24]

Chapter 11

∞

Controversy in Electroshock

When European totalitarianism drove many psychiatrists to the West, these men and women brought with them their experience with both psychoanalysis and electroshock. The psychoanalysts flourished in America, and their leaders were promoted high in the ranks of academic psychiatry. They soon exerted great influence on clinical practice and teaching. In the 1960s, most departments of psychiatry in the United States were headed by analysts.

But philosophic squabbles arose between the psychoanalysts of the Freudian school and those of the neo-Freudian schools, as well as with those relying on biological treatments. Public arguments about differences in philosophy and practice brought psychoanalysts into conflict with more traditional therapists who saw the merits of somatic therapies. Such conflicts were pushed off center stage by the introduction of psychoactive drugs in the late 1950s. Both somatic treatments and psychoanalysis faded; the disciples of psychopharmacology began to take the lead in clinical practice, education, and research.

The sterling promises of the new drugs soon became tarnished, however, as patients failed to recover despite repeated medication trials. The few clinicians who had used ECT returned to it and found that the drug-resistant cases could be effectively treated. Successes of ECT after medication failures were known by the mid-1960s, and by the early 1970s interest in ECT had revived.

The time for the reconsideration of ECT was inopportune because many saw the forced treatment of the mentally ill as another example of abuse of the power of the state. Disgust with the treatment of the mentally ill had already surfaced during World War II with the publication of *The Mentally Ill in America* and *The Shame of the States*, both by Albert Deutsch.[1] Deutsch depicted the sordid conditions under which the mentally ill were cared for in state mental health facilities and was vehement in his condemnation of lobotomy and electroshock used against the wishes of patients. He was encouraged and supported by the American Foundation for Mental Hygiene, a foundation started by Clifford Beers, a former patient who had described his recovery from psychosis in the acclaimed 1908 account *A Mind That Found Itself.*[2]

A graphic example of abuse is depicted in Ken Kesey's book *One Flew Over the Cuckoo's Nest* and in the 1975 film based on the novel. The protagonist is subjected to both electroshock and, at the end, to bilateral lobotomy against his will. The unavoidable message is that electroshock and lobotomy are cruelties.

Public attention focused mainly on lobotomy, but few critics distinguished it from electroshock. The damnation of one was called down upon both. Complaints that ECT was used excessively and inappropriately on children and adolescents further fueled the opposition to its reinstatement.[3]

A second impediment to the revival was its reputation for being a painful, inhumane treatment. When it was introduced, electroshock was given without anesthetic, and patients approached each treatment with anxiety, dread, and panic. Some patients sustained fractures; some died. Anesthesia, muscle relaxation, and hyperoxygenation were answers to the problems, but they were not accepted as routine measures until the mid-1950s, after 20 years of unmodified ECT.

Unmodified treatments did harm memory, so much so that memory loss came to be seen as an essential part of the treatment. It was this effect that remained in the public's mind as the main outcome of the treatment. Few in the public and in mental health practice were aware that the treatment had changed dramatically and that the negative effect on memory had been sharply reduced by the technical changes of continuous oxygenation (1953), unilateral electrode placement (1971), brief-pulse energy currents (1976), and seizure-duration monitoring (1982). These changes had become integral to "modified ECT."

A third impediment to ECT's revival was the enmity expressed by psychoanalysts. At the end of World War II, the Freudian philosophy had moved beyond the academy to the marketplace, and a patient of a Freudian analyst found he had a special cachet among the nation's intelligentsia and its artists. From a discipline limited to the care of the insane in state-supported wards for the mentally ill, psychiatry had become a socially accepted item of parlor conversation and an interesting discipline for physicians. Psychoanalytic principles were accepted as a source of ideas for political and social change. A greater tolerance and permissiveness in child-rearing was one example, represented by the almost universal acceptance of Dr. Benjamin Spock's writings, based on Freudian psychoanalytic principles, as a guide for child care.[4]

The benefits of both the psychological and the somatic treatments were overstated. For many mental disorders it was unclear which treatment, if any, was appropriate. While psychoanalysts focused their attention on patients who had neurotic symptoms, with facility in expressing their thoughts, and a life and career, some analysts, instead, sought patients with schizophrenia, manic-depressive insanity, and the more severe delusional disorders. They claimed that their methods would raise unconscious conflicts to consciousness and that the patient, in "working through" these conflicts, would remove the cause of his mental disorder. Case reports were accepted as dogma, and many patients were subjected to unnecessary and often disastrous periods of verbal therapy that only delayed their recovery.[5] The same authors deprecated the efforts of psychiatrists who emphasized the use of drugs and electroshock, and accused them of burying dynamic conflicts further by impairing memory and deepening repression.

The hostility between disciplines intensified after the war, when psychoanalysts established the Group for the Advancement of Psychiatry, a society whose aim was to establish psychodynamic practice as the core discipline of psychiatry. The members sought leadership positions in the American Psychiatric Association and on medical school campuses, but the challenge to their position in psychiatric practice was the continuing reliance of patients on electroshock. The members of GAP considered such use a direct philosophic and economic affront. Their first public action was the wide distribution, on May 15, 1947, of a one-page broadside listing its objections to the use of electroshock.[6] The paper concluded:

> Your committee feels that overemphasis and unjustified use of electro-shock therapy short-circuits the training and experience which is essential in modern dynamic psychiatry.
>
> Abuses in the use of electro-shock therapy are sufficiently widespread and dangerous to justify consideration of a cam-

paign of professional education in the limitations of this technique, and perhaps even to justify instituting certain measures of control.

The profession reacted by demanding a public withdrawal. An apology was issued, but psychoanalysts continued to express their hostility.[7] The antipathy, also voiced by their followers in psychology, social work, and child and adolescent psychiatry, remains the principal cause of the remaining distrust of electroshock.[8]

The conflict within the profession has had many consequences. Practitioners who sought to bridge the two disciplines were rejected by both sides. The qualifying board examination in neurology and psychiatry, one test that originally certified practitioners in both disciplines, was divided into two certifying examinations. The disciplines now have separate teaching and clinical practice requisites and procedures, and the care of many patients with mental and brain disorders unfortunately falls between the two. Most egregious, however, is the inexcusable failure of academic psychiatrists to consider electroshock as a core discipline in their teaching or in the care of their patients, a neglect that encourages poor treatment, prolonged illness, even suicide.[9]

Restrictions on Electroshock

The introduction of psychotropic drugs, and the national advertising campaigns proclaiming their merits, led the public to assume that none of the somatic treatments—not lobotomy, insulin coma, or electroshock—warranted continued use. Harrowing tales of patients treated against their will initiated legislative interdiction of lobotomy and electroshock in some states in the early 1970s. The laws forced psychiatrists to question whether the treatments were worth salvaging, and under what conditions their use should be encouraged. But lobotomy had already been superseded by psychotropic drugs, so no scientific reviews were undertaken. The results of insulin coma had been so poor that it had also been abandoned.[10]

The assessments of electroshock and drugs, undertaken earlier, had established that the drugs mimicked the efficacy of electroshock. That, together with the greater ease of use and lesser expense, certainly influenced psychiatrists to forgo electroshock therapy and devote their practices to psychotropic drugs and psychotherapy. Though some patients were not helped by the drugs and might have benefited from ECT, the legal proscription of electroshock made it difficult for psychiatrists to call on the treatment. When a number of psychiatrists raised questions about the reintroduction of electroshock, reassessments of its merits and risks were once again undertaken. Between 1972 and 1985, government agencies, commissions authorized by national societies, and individual practitioners evaluated the treatment. All were sufficiently impressed to advocate its continued use.[11]

Proposed restrictions on psychiatric practice by the Massachusetts legislature in 1971 led the commissioner of mental health to establish a task force of the Massachusetts Psychiatric Society. The members concluded that the indications for ECT were well defined for patients with affective disorders, but they regarded its benefits for patients with schizophrenia and for prepubertal children as unproven. They cautioned against extensive courses of treatments, since there had been little study of their adverse effects. The commissioner then issued regulations that defined the indications for ECT, required adherence to reporting and consent procedures, and limited the numbers of treatments that could be given to an individual patient in any one year.[12] His action forestalled legislative restrictions of the treatment.

In 1973 the California legislature also sought to interdict the use of electroshock, lobotomy, and psychotropic drugs. As the proposed law progressed through the legislative process, objections to the use of psychoactive drugs were dropped, largely because the public was aghast at the possible restriction of the popular tranquilizers Miltown and Valium. Both ECT and lobotomy were interdicted, but the law was challenged in court and enjoined as an illegal restriction on medical practice. The legislature revised the law to set consent and reporting requirements and to limit the use of ECT in patients under the age of 12. This law was upheld in the court as within the protective powers of the state, and the availability and the use of ECT in California has consequently been tightly narrowed.[13]

Other states also restricted the use of ECT. In 1976 the Tennessee legislature limited the use of ECT in patients under 14, and in 1977, its use in Colorado was restricted in those under 16. The

Texas legislature in 1993 banned the administration of ECT to patients under 16 and required practitioners to report to the state all treatments given to patients.

The ECT-reporting requirements provide a picture of actual practice. A 1998 report of 15,240 treatments administered over 19 months between 1993 and 1995 in Texas indicated that almost all the patients were white (88 percent), two-thirds were women, and half were elderly.[14] Nearly all the treatments were given in academic and private mental hospitals, with only one of 13 state-funded mental institutions providing ECT. Almost all, 97.5 percent, were voluntary patients who gave their own consent for the treatment, 1.5 percent were consenting involuntary patients, and 0.9 percent were patients with guardian or court consent. The law requires the reporting of any untoward events within 14 days of treatment; no adverse events were reported in conjunction with the actual administration of treatments, but eight deaths occurred within the two-week reporting period. An elderly patient with a history of multiple heart attacks and systemic treatment died in the recovery room; he had been receiving outpatient ECT on a maintenance schedule for many years. The other seven deaths were unrelated to the treatments. Fewer than 6 percent of licensed Texas psychiatrists administered the treatments.

California's laws similarly restrict the use of ECT.[15] The treatment is not available in the state-managed hospitals or in many of the smaller community hospitals that serve the uninsured, members of minority groups, and the more severely ill.

Antipsychiatry actions

In the years after World War II, psychiatry became the target of two men in the United States, Thomas Szasz and L. Ron Hubbard. Szasz, a Hungarian psychiatrist exiled by Nazism, was appointed professor at the medical school of the State University of New York in Syracuse. From this vantage point, he excoriated psychiatrists and their use of psychotropic drugs, asserting that mental illness was a myth created by professionals acting as agents of the state to intimidate and incarcerate citizens.[16] He characterized psychiatric treatments, especially drugs and electroshock, as an abuse of state power and decried any treatment of mental disorders, alleging that individuals had the right to believe what they wished. His statements, perhaps indicating an overreaction to his experience with fascism and communism, attracted a small but vociferous cadre of active anti-psychiatrists. Szasz's attacks on psychiatric practice, taken up by his disciples in child and adolescent psychiatry, psychology, social work, and religion, discouraged patients from considering psychiatric treatments other than some brand of psychotherapy. His student Peter Breggin became a professional critic of the use of biological treatments, testifying before state legislatures and Congress in favor of laws to prohibit their use. He has written diatribes against conventional psychiatry and actively supports malpractice suits against psychiatrists.[17] His personal experience with electroshock is limited to his training in Syracuse and Boston in the 1970s.

Similar attacks on psychiatric practice occurred in Europe. Ronald Laing (1967) in Great Britain, Michel Foucault (1965) in France, and Franco Basaglia in Italy argued that mental illness was a social phenomenon, secondary to economic and political problems, not related to biological causes. Psychiatric practices based on medical interventions were so distorted by these critics that in 1978 Italy closed the country's large mental institutions, forcing families and communities to assume the responsibility of caring for the mentally ill.[18] This experiment was recognized as a failure only when the mentally ill flooded Italian city streets and overwhelmed their families' capabilities to care for them.

When L. Ron Hubbard established the social movement known as the Church of Scientology, he made the psychiatric care of the mentally ill his target. He argued that the use of psychotropic medications, electroshock, and lobotomy are immoral and damaging to the brain, and that no person would voluntarily agree to a treatment that might alter the mind. His international following condemns biological treatments throughout the world, and his followers are the most active antagonists of psychiatric practice. The Church of Scientology has several publishing outlets, using the imprimaturs Citizens Commission on Human Rights, Bridge Publications, New Era Publications, and Freedom Publications.[19] Among their widely distributed publications are *Psychiatry Destroys Minds, Psychiatry's Betrayal, Psychiatry Victimizing the Elderly, Psychiatry Destroying Religion, Psychiatry Destroying*

Morals, and *Psychiatry Manipulates Creativity,* most of which are sent free to medical students and psychiatric residents.

An account published in *The New Yorker* in 1974 of an alleged case of brain damage following ECT strengthened the anti-psychiatry movement. Berton Roueché, a prominent medical writer, told the story of a federal government economist named Marilyn Rice. She had pain in her teeth that was not relieved by extensive dental care; eventually all her teeth were removed. When the pain persisted, she sought psychiatric help but got no relief from psychotherapy or medicines. At that point, she was referred for ECT. After it was administered, her dental pains disappeared, but she complained that all memory of her past and her profession had also disappeared. She claimed she needed a laborious relearning in order to function at all. Eventually, she retired from government service and then started publicly attacking ECT. She spoke at psychiatric conferences, appeared before state legislatures, and wrote harshly critical letters about psychiatrists and psychiatry. She established the Committee Against Assault in Psychiatry, a vocal antipsychiatry group that still seeks public attention.

Attacks on ECT continue to be featured on television and radio talk shows and in newspaper articles.[20] A series of four articles published in 1995 in the national newspaper *USA Today,* written in conjunction with the debates in the Texas legislature to outlaw ECT, presents a particularly egregious example. It alleged that psychiatrists resort to treating the elderly and children with ECT when other means would have done as well. Practitioners use ECT because of financial incentives, not clinical judgment, the series said. It also claimed that death rates were much higher than were reported in the psychiatric literature.[21]

While many public figures acknowledge having been treated for their dependence on alcohol and sedative drugs, for breast cancer, and even for AIDS, few acknowledge that they were treated with electroshock. The tragic experience of Senator Thomas Eagleton, who had been named the candidate for the vice presidency on the Democratic ticket in 1972, is well known. He was forced to withdraw when the press turned his experience with ECT into front-page news. Ernest Hemingway's experience with alcoholism, depression, and attempted suicide led to a course of ECT, which resolved his depression for some time. When the author's alcoholism persisted and another depressive episode led to a successful suicide, the episode was trumpeted as an example of failed ECT. The pianist Vladimir Horowitz retired from public performances on numerous occasions, presumably because of depression. After his death, his obituary noted that he had had a successful course of ECT before his triumphant final return to the stage and his successful performances at the White House and in Russia and Japan. The recent Australian film *Shine* depicted the story of David Helfgott, a pianist who suffered a psychotic episode early in his career and returned to a more normal life after a course of ECT. The film presented the tardive dyskinesia and episodic explosive and repetitive speech that marked his condition. Doctors recognize that these motor signs are clearly the result of extensive treatment with neuroleptic drugs, not the consequence of electroshock. Other public figures who have acknowledged successful experience with ECT are the TV commentator Dick Cavett and Roland Kohloff, a tympanist with the New York Philharmonic Orchestra.

Professional response

In 1975, following passage of the restrictive California legislation, the American Psychiatric Association established the Task Force on Electroconvulsive Therapy, similar to the one that had been established in Massachusetts.[22] The task force members surveyed the use of ECT by members of the association, reviewed the published accounts, and held public hearings in order to get a clear image of contemporary ECT practice. Their report, endorsed by the trustees of the association in 1978, supported the use of ECT for patients with major depressive disorders and with mania, and particularly for those whom psychotropic drugs had not helped. Most important was the panel's recommendation of a formal consent procedure to ensure that ECT was administered only to consenting patients. The panel also issued detailed descriptions of treatment techniques. The report was adopted by many hospitals in establishing standards for ECT practice.

A survey of ECT practice in Great Britain was undertaken in 1980. Assessors observed the actual clinical practice in a hundred sites and evaluated the views of members of the Royal College of Psychiatrists, heads of psychiatric facilities, and some general practitioners. Their conclusions about indications, risks, and guidelines for practice were similar to those in the American report.

The authors also found, however, that in some parts of the nation, more than half the ECT devices were obsolete, and that in 40 percent of the sites the instruments were not properly maintained.[23] When the report was brought to the attention of the editors of *The Lancet*, a highly esteemed weekly international journal of medicine, the editors wrote a review titled "ECT in Britain: A Shameful State of Affairs," in which they concluded:

> Every British psychiatrist should read this report and feel ashamed and worried about the state of British psychiatry. If ECT is ever legislated against or falls into disuse it will not be because it is an ineffective or dangerous treatment; it will be because psychiatrists have failed to supervise and monitor its use adequately. It is not ECT which has brought psychiatry into disrepute. Psychiatry has done just that for ECT.[24]

Although the National Health Service did authorize expenditures to improve the practice of ECT, a follow-up survey, conducted in 1992 by one of the original surveyors, found ECT practice to have changed very little.[25] More recent essays find the training in ECT to be still inadequate.[26]

A similar survey in Ireland found the use of ECT and the professional opinions to be similar to those in Great Britain, with the use and numbers of treatments in a series slightly higher.[27] A Canadian Queen's Counsel commission examined the use of ECT in the province of Ontario in response to public demands that ECT be condemned as "brain-damaging." The commission "favored continuing the availability of ECT . . . [and] recognized the necessity of extensive safeguards relating to the use of ECT based on sound legal, ethical and medical practices."[28]

The recurrent outcry against ECT led the U.S. National Institutes of Health and of Mental Health to convene a consensus development conference from June 10 to 12, 1985, to address questions of efficacy, risks, and adverse effects, appropriateness of treatment, optimal administration, and directions for research in ECT. The "controversial" nature of the treatment was emphasized, yet the panel found ECT demonstrably effective for severe psychiatric disorders. It recommended a continuing consultative process for consent, additional research, a national survey of practice (which was not done), and the development of national guidelines for practice.[29]

Support for the continued use of electroshock also came from the American Medical Association[30] and several national mental health associations, including the National Mental Health Association, the National Depressive and Manic-Depressive Association (NDMDA), and the National Alliance for the Mentally Ill (NAMI).[31]

The renewed use of ECT was noted as well in the press. In 1987, the *New York Times* discussed it in an article titled "Shock Therapy: Return to Respectability," which alluded to the legislative and antipsychiatry controversies and also related the successful applications and safety of the treatment.[32] An article in *New York* magazine in 1994, titled "When Prozac Fails . . . Electroshock Works," reflected the reporter's ambivalence from the start: "It's still popularly feared and reviled. But these days it's kinder and gentler—and widely used. Electroshock is jolting thousands of patients out of suicidal depressions."[33]

Questions about the mode of action of ECT stimulated interest. How could seizures bring about beneficial effects in behavior? In 1972, with support from the National Institute of Mental Health, psychiatrists at a conference on the biological effects of electroshock reviewed the effects of seizures on brain electrophysiology, chemistry, and memory. No theory of ECT's action emerged.[34] In 1985, psychiatrists at an international conference in New York reviewed the research issues that had received attention during the previous decade.[35] Those attending the conference concluded that how ECT works still remained a mystery.

To support greater communication among ECT researchers, I established the quarterly journal *Convulsive Therapy* in 1985. The American Psychiatric Association established a second Task Force on Electroconvulsive Therapy in 1988 to update the standards of clinical practice.[36]

In 1991, the National Institutes of Health held a conference on the recognition and treatment of depression in the elderly. The consensus was that ECT filled an important role in the treatment of depression in elderly adults; that the evidence for short-term efficacy of ECT is strong; and that relapse after effective ECT is frequent, requiring further study of alternate treatment strategies, including continuation ECT. The panel found that ECT, despite its efficacy, is generally underused by, or unavailable to, the elderly.[37]

Consequences of controversy

The controversies have taken a toll. The availability of ECT is uneven and sparse. Many facilities licensed to treat the mentally ill are not equipped to deliver the treatment. And so few psychiatrists are skilled in electroshock therapy that patients in many parts of the country don't have access to the treatment.[38]

The techniques of ECT are meant to be taught in postgraduate psychiatric residency programs, along with psychotherapy and psychopharmacology, but few programs offer the training. As a consequence, practitioners who seek to develop their skills in ECT must do so in continuing-medical-education programs. These generally run from one to five days, too brief a time to establish a relationship with patients, work through possible problems in treatment, and observe the changes in the subject's mental state. Observation is deemed so essential for other psychiatric treatments, especially psychotherapy and pharmacotherapy, that psychiatrists cannot be certified as specialists unless they have had such experience. Yet practitioners of electroshock are left to develop their experience while treating their first patients. No one examines the practitioners' skills in the complex techniques of ECT.[39] The national certification boards in psychiatry and neurology ignore it, setting neither minimal standards for education nor prerequisites for certification. In fact, practitioners in ECT are self-declared. Few hospitals question the competence of the physicians they allow to use their facilities for ECT.[40] A similar indifference to training is reported in Great Britain.[41]

In those states where ECT is legally restricted, even patients who have accepted the recommendation for treatment are unable to get it unless they uproot themselves. The restrictions not only limit the use of ECT in defined populations; they change the perception of the treatment. After all, if the government interdicts its use, it must be dangerous.

It is this attitude that inflicts on patients prolonged periods of illness, chronic illness, or death. In the procedures in which psychiatric insurers allow payments for psychiatric treatment, ECT is an option that comes late in the course of the illness, usually after one medication trial after another has failed. Such an attitude makes it impossible for the managed care insurers, including Medicare and Medicaid, to do other than ignore ECT or to relegate it to the treatment of suicidal patients or to those who have suffered far too long.

Chapter 12

∞

Electroshock in the 1990s

Within the past decade, clinical and research interest in ECT has revived. The resurgence has been most marked in the United States, where the greatest efforts are under way to improve its safety and its efficacy.[1] Psychiatrists in other countries have sought to reintroduce ECT, but its use varies widely. ECT is an accepted part of psychiatric practice in the Scandinavian countries, Great Britain, Ireland, Australia, and New Zealand, and usage is similar to that in the United States. A stigma attached to ECT limits its use in Germany, Japan, Italy, and the Netherlands to a few academic medical centers. Low reimbursement rates hamper its use in Canada and Japan, and also affect its availability in the United States. The unavailability of modern equipment and the expense of the medicines for anesthesia prevent its use in Africa, Asia, and Eastern Europe, and many patients in these countries who do receive it are subjected to unmodified ECT, such as was delivered in the 1930s and 1940s.

ECT is mainly a treatment for hospitalized patients, although many institutions are developing programs for outpatient ECT. The equipment and trained personnel are, for the most part, in the academic hospitals. Academic leaders recognize the merits of the treatment; some even encourage research and teaching. ECT is ignored by the research scientists at the National Institute of Mental Health. Few of the state, federal, or Veterans Administration hospitals provide ECT, and where it is available its use is infrequent. While 8 percent to 12 percent of adult inpatients at academic hospitals receive ECT, fewer than 0.2 percent of adults at nonacademic centers do.[2] Such a discrepancy reflects the continuing social stigma and philosophical bias against electroshock. Before the federal Medicare and the Hill-Burton legislative acts of the 1960s opened access for all patients to any hospital facility, such discrepancies may have been common. But now that the nation has adopted an open-admission policy to its psychiatric facilities, the discrepancy is unjustified. It is shameful that many agencies licensed to treat the mentally ill lack the facilities to give the treatment.[3]

Effects of research on practice

When ECT was revived in the late 1970s, the principal concern was its effects on cognition and memory. Unilateral ECT won favor with many practitioners after demonstrations that it reduced effects on memory.[4] But other practitioners reported that unilateral ECT required more treatments than, and was not as effective as, bilateral ECT. The seizures in unilateral ECT were often brief, with poorly defined EEG seizure patterns. Studies of the interaction of electrode placement, energy dosing, and current form show that unilateral treatments, even with precise energy dosing, are less efficient than bilateral ECT.[5] As a result, bilateral ECT is now preferred. When unilateral ECT is considered, its use includes precise energy dosing. Sinusoidal currents elicited unnecessarily high degrees of EEG and memory effects, compared with brief pulse square-wave currents, so the former have now been discarded.[6]

We have learned that monitoring the motor seizure is not sufficient to measure the adequacy of an individual treatment, so we now look to EEG measures as more reliable indices.[7] By recording and displaying the seizure EEG, we rely on the seizure characteristics as a guide to an effective treatment. Practitioners depend more on these characteristics than on criteria based on the motor convulsion and the change in heart rate as measures of beneficial treatment.[8]

The interseizure EEG has stimulated research interest. Studies in 1957 had shown that a good clinical response in ECT depended on the slowing of the frequencies in the interseizure EEG.[9] The observation was confirmed in 1972 and again in 1996, and the interseizure EEG is once again used as a guide to an effective course of treatment.[10]

The indications for ECT have been broadened. As we have seen, it has gone from being a last resort for unresponsive depressed and suicidal patients to being a treatment option for patients with delusional depression, mania, schizophrenia, and catatonia. ECT can also be useful in patients with parkinsonism and those suffering from neuroleptic drug toxicity. Treatment can be safely given in the presence of complex systemic disorders and mental retardation.

Yet research on ECT is limited. Most of the research is directed at determining which treatment—medication or continuation ECT—can best maintain the benefits of a course of ECT in patients with severe depression. Some scientists still believe that sophisticated brain-imaging methods will find evidence of persistent brain dysfunction after ECT. So far, such studies have yielded no new information about mental illness or about ECT. Others seek the benefits of ECT without a seizure by the use of rapid magnetic pulses instead of electrical ones. The method, called "rapid transcranial magnetic stimulation" (rTMS), has yet to be proven of benefit.

Future of electroshock

Psychiatric care in the United States is in such turmoil that the problem of restoring the availability of electroshock seems nearly insignificant. American psychiatry lacks the leaders to stand up to the pharmaceutical industry and the managed care executives who are taking ever larger portions of the financial resources allocated to treating mental illness. State legislatures are cutting funds for mental health care, urging their mental hospital administrators to reduce patient admissions and shorten durations of stay. The state mental hospitals, which served as the ultimate haven for the mentally ill, are being closed and patients are being consigned to a motley collection of inadequate substitutions. The nonthreatening and passive homeless are on the streets; those who are more ill go in and out of the revolving doors of community centers and emergency wards or to hospitals equipped only for short-term care. Those who fall between end up in halfway houses and adult homes.

At one time the states supported research centers that were the jewels of the nation's mental health activities. Few institutes are still supported by the states, and even these are forced to compete for larger portions of their budgets from federal resources and private charity.

Academic researchers depend on industry to support increasing portions of their salaries. Industry sponsorship has taken over major aspects of the training of psychiatric residents by providing funds for lectures and seminars at medical schools and hospitals, and for national and international meetings. Industry employees organize carefully crafted symposia, and the ensuing discussions are published as supplements to freely distributed psychiatric journals.[11] The opportunity for independent assessment and open dialogue about the efficacy and safety of psychoactive drugs, and especially comparisons with other treatments such as electroshock, has been virtually eliminated.

The leaders of the lay agencies that speak for the mentally ill are confused, torn between the promises of an industry hawking its products, state mental health agencies seeking to self-destruct, and managed care companies striving to limit expenditures for the care of the mentally ill. The lay agencies are sensitive to the stigma of electroshock and avoid mention of it for fear of losing members and financial support. For that reason, they do not encourage state and municipal legislatures to provide the treatment.

In this turmoil, few psychiatrists speak up in behalf of electroshock for their patients. The two U.S. manufacturers who make modern ECT devices and support educational efforts are too small to do more than survive. Although their new devices have highly sophisticated EEG-recording capabilities that can monitor electroshock treatments with great precision, these manufacturers can do little to ensure that their instruments are properly used.

In the brouhaha over the revival of ECT in the 1970s, the anti-ECT lobby tried to persuade the FDA to limit the sale and use of ECT devices in the United States. Their claim was that the devices were unsafe. In the early 1980s the FDA ruled that the devices in use were safe and reliable. The devices delivered energies with a fixed maximum under standard conditions, a maximum that had been set arbitrarily.[12] Patients' seizure thresholds, however, rise with age, and many of the elderly need higher energies for effective treatment.[13] The device manufacturers developed such devices, but when they applied to the FDA for modification of the standards, they were turned down and could not sell their equipment. The devices now sold in the United States are inadequate for effective treatment of some patients.[14] Since the higher-energy devices are sold in the rest of the world, we have the awkward situation that patients in Canada, Europe, and Australia are being effectively treated while we in this country fail in treating some patients with similar conditions.[15]

There is one opportunity on the economic horizon for a broader recognition of the merits of electroshock.[16] The duration of inpatient treatment for patients receiving electroshock seems to be longer than for those receiving other treatments. But patients come to ECT after drug trials, often many trials, have failed. If the duration of inpatient care of patients given ECT is estimated from the day of the decision to use ECT, it is shorter and the costs are lower than the costs for psychotropic drugs. In one academic general hospital, of 19 depressed patients treated with ECT alone, the average hospital stay averaged 41 days, and for the 55 patients treated with tricyclic antidepressants (TCA) alone, the average stay was 55 days. The longest stay was for patients first treated with TCA and, when those failed, with ECT—an average length of stay of 71 days. The estimated cost of the stay for ECT treatment was $20,000 and for TCA alone it was $26,500, a savings of $6,500 for ECT over TCA.[17] The same financial advantage is found when outpatient ECT is prescribed.[18]

A study of patients discharged from general hospitals with a principal diagnosis of depressive disorder found that the initiation of ECT within five days of admission leads to shorter and less costly inpatient treatment than for those treated with drugs alone or delayed ECT.[19] Other studies found that the antidepressant effects of ECT occur earlier and are more robust than those of antidepressant drugs.[20]

For the present, few managed care insurers recognize the merits of ECT, either as a relief for their insured ill patients or as a financial benefit to their shareholders.[21] Payment for ECT is rarely approved for a patient with schizophrenia, so that patient must endure one drug trial after another. The most specious arguments are made about patients seen as catatonic, where neuroleptic drug trials are required, despite the evidence that neuroleptic drugs may precipitate the more acute state of neuroleptic malignant syndrome (NMS).

As managed care organizations assume a greater role in medical care, they reduce costs by limiting the conditions for which payments will be made, cutting professional fees and negotiating cheaper hospital costs. Once these measures have squeezed out of the system all the "excess" costs they can, the demand for the most efficient treatments will gain support. The advantages of ECT over medication should promote its greater use. Such an effect is already apparent in the expanding number of institutions seeking to develop qualified ECT facilities, in the interest of practitioners in obtaining education credits for ECT, and in the overt inclusion of electroshock as a valid treatment in algorithms now recommended for depression.[22]

Many object to the revival of ECT by reminding others of the problems with electroshock when it was first introduced; at the time it was virtually the only effective treatment for the mentally ill. Such criticism is wholly unwarranted today; it is no more reasonable than to speak of the excesses in tonsillectomy, hysterectomy, pallidotomy, insulin coma, and lobotomy that marked the enthusiastic reception of those procedures in earlier decades. Our appreciation of electroshock must be based on its present practice. We call on it because it is effective, often more so than alternate treatments, and because modern practice has made it safe.

Appendix 1

∞

Diagnoses in Which ECT
Is Considered Effective**

Major depression	
single episode	[296.2x]*
recurrent	[296.3x]*
Bipolar major depression	
depressed	[296.5x]*
mixed	[296.6x]*
not otherwise specified	[296.70]*
Mania (bipolar disorder)	
mania	[296.4x]*
mixed type	[296.6x]*
not otherwise specified	[296.70]*
Atypical psychosis	[298.90]
Schizophrenia	
catatonic	[295.2x]
schizophreniform	[295.40]
schizo-affective	[295.70]
Catatonia	
Schizophrenia, catatonic type	[295.2x]
Catatonic disorder due to medical condition	[293.89]
Malignant catatonia	[293.89]
Neuroleptic malignant syndrome	[333.92]
Delirium	
Due to a general medical condition	[293.0]
Due to substance intoxication [specify substance]	[291.8x]

*Especially when associated with delusions
**According to the American Psychiatric Association's *Diagnostic and Statistical Manual of Mental Disorders*, Edition IV, 1994

Appendix 2

∞

Diagnoses in Which ECT Is Considered Ineffective

Dementia and amnestic disorders	[293.0, 290.xx, 294.xx]
Substance-related disorders	[303.xx, 291, x, 304.x, 292.x]
Anxiety and somatiform disorders	[300.xx]
Factitious disorders	[300.xx]
Dissociative disorders	[300.1x, 300.6]
Sexual dysfunctions	[302.xx, 625.8, 608.89, 607.84, 608.89, 625.8]
Sleep disorders	[307.xx, 780.xx]
Impulse disorders	[312.3x]
Adjustment disorders	[309.xx]
Personality disorders	[301.xx]

Appendix 3

∞

Sample Consent Form for Electrotherapy

I, _____, M.D. (and _____, M.D.) recommend electroconvulsive therapy for your present mental symptoms. These treatments have been given to thousands of mentally ill patients since 1938, with many improvements in the treatments and greater success in helping patients since then.

Treatments are given in the mornings before breakfast, in a specially equipped treatment room. You will be attended by an anesthetist, a nurse, and a psychiatrist.

A needle will be placed in your vein (like you may have had when samples were taken for blood tests) and an anesthetic will be injected. You will become drowsy and fall asleep. Other medicines will be given to relax your muscles. The anesthetist will help you breathe with pure oxygen through a mask.

The treatment is given while you are asleep. Momentary electric currents are passed through electrodes on the scalp to stimulate the brain. A grand-mal seizure and muscular contractions for up to two minutes follow; with proper relaxation, the contractions are barely measurable.

The treatments take only a few minutes. You are then moved to the recovery room where you will wake up as after a deep sleep. You may feel groggy, and will probably have muscular aches, similar to those after exercising, and a headache. You will return to your room, usually within an hour of the treatment. You will be given your breakfast and spend the rest of the morning on the ward with your nurse or attendant.

Treatments are given every other day for up to 12 treatments. Many patients improve rapidly and require fewer treatments, some require more than 12, but these would not be given without another discussion with you and your family.

The treatment has risks. The treatments are given in a room where special equipment and supplies for your protection are available. Patients often become confused, and may not know where they are when they awaken. This may be frightening, but the confusion usually disappears within a few hours. Memory for recent events, mainly for the period of illness and the treatment, may be disturbed. Dates, names of friends, public events, telephone numbers, and addresses may be difficult to recall. In most patients, the memory difficulty is gone within four weeks after the last treatment; but rarely, the problems remain for months, and even years. Death is a rare complication occurring no more frequently than death in mothers giving spontaneous birth. Equally uncommon with modern anesthesia are bone fractures, broken or lost teeth, and spontaneous seizures after the treatment is over, but these may occur.

You may discontinue the treatments at any time, although you will be encouraged to continue until an adequate course is completed.

I, _____, have read this description of the treatments and these have been explained to me by _____.

I agree to have the treatments and understand that Dr. _____ will be the physician in charge of my treatment.

Dated: _____ Agreed: _____

Witness: _____ Relationship to Patient: _____

Appendix 4

Medicines

Popular Name	Scientific Name	Use
Amidate	etomidate	anesthetic
Amytal	amobarbital	anesthetic/sedative
Anapsine	droperidol	anesthetic
Anectine	succinylcholine	muscle relaxant
Artane	trihexyphenidil	antiparkinson
Ativan	lorazepam	sedative
atropine	atropine	anticholinergic
Benadryl	diphenhydramine	sedative
Brevital	methohexital	anesthetic
Capoten	captopril	anti-hypertensive
Clozaril	clozapine	atypical antipsychotic
Cogentin	benztropine	antiparkinson
Coumadin	warfarin	anticoagulant
Dentrium	dantrolene	muscle relaxant
Depakote	divalproex	anticonvulsant
Diprivan	propofol	anesthetic
Elavil	amitriptyline	antidepressant (TCA)
Haldol	haloperidol	antipsychotic
Ketalar	ketamine	anesthetic
Klonipin	clonazepam	sedative
Lanoxin	digoxin	cardiac stimulant
Lithobid	lithium	antimanic
Metrazol	pentylenetetrazol	induces seizures
Miltown	meprobamate	anxiolytic
Moban	molindone	antipsychotic
Nardil	phenelzine	antidepressant (MAOI)
Navane	thiothixene	antipsychotic
Norpamin	desipramine	antidepressant (TCA)
Pamelor	nortriptyline	antidepressant (TCA)
Parlodel	bromocriptine	dopamine agonist
Paxil	paroxetine	antidepressant (SSRI)
Pentothal	thiopental	anesthetic

Prolixin	fluphenazine	antipsychotic
Prozac	fluoxetine	antidepressant (SSRI)
Risperdal	risperidone	atypical antipsychotic
Robinul	glycopyrrolate	anticholinergic
Romazicon	flumazenil	benzodiazepine antagonist
Sinemet	*l*-dopa	dopamine agonist
Sinequan	doxepin	antidepressant (TCA)
Tegretol	carbamazepine	anticonvulsant
Thorazine	chlorpromazine	antipsychotic
Tofranil	imipramine	antidepressant (TCA)
Trilafon	perphenazine	antipsychotic
Valium	diazepam	sedative
Versed	midazolam	sedative
Xanax	alprazolam	anxiolytic
Zoloft	sertraline	antidepressant (SSRI)
Zyprexa	olanzapine	atypical antipsychotic

Notes

Preface

1. Some accounts have been published in medical literature. The articles illustrate ECT in patients with neuroleptic malignant syndrome (Greenberg and Gujavarty, 1985; Fricchione et al., 1990), toxic serotonin syndrome (Fink, 1996b), intracranial lesions (Greenberg, Mofson, Fink, 1988; Greenberg et al., 1986), severe anemia (LaGrone, 1990), pseudodementia (Bright-Long and Fink, 1993), and auricular fibrillation (Petrides and Fink, 1996a). Our experience with ECT in adolescent patients (Moise and Petrides, 1996), schizophrenia (Gujavarty, Greenberg, Fink, 1987; Fink and Sackeim, 1996), mental retardation (Thuppal and Fink, in press), and the elderly (Greenberg and Fink, 1990) has also been described.

Chapter 1: What Is Electroshock?

1. Continuation ECT is a feature of modern practice. In an index course, treatments continue for four to six months. If the illness recurs, ECT may be given for up to a year. In rare cases, treatments have been continued for years.
2. Fink, 1997b.
3. Faber and Trimble, 1991; Fink, 1988.
4. APA, 1990, pp. 7, 49–50.
5. Abrams, 1998.

Chapter 2: The Patient's Experience

1. Fink 1986a,b.
2. A formal consent procedure, the first in psychiatric practice, was recommended for ECT in the report of the first Task Force on Electroconvulsive Therapy of the American Psychiatric Association (APA, 1978).
3. Psychoactive drugs have many risks, some persistent. For antipsy-

chotic drugs, tardive dyskinesia, tardive dystonia, parkinsonism, and the neuroleptic malignant syndrome are frequent. For the atypical antipsychotic Clozaril, blood dyscrasia is a risk that warrants weekly or biweekly blood examinations. Lithium is associated with tremor, diarrhea, and confusion. Antidepressant drugs are accompanied by cardiac risks, including the risk of sudden death, confusion, and delirium.

4. Booklets are available from the National Institute of Mental Health (Sargent, 1986), the MECTA Corporation (1988), and Somatics Inc. (Abrams and Swartz, 1991). The videotapes are cited as Fink, 1986b; Grunhaus, 1988; Royal College of Psychiatrists, 1994.

5. Unfortunately, many judges are ill acquainted with the advantages of electroshock and will not order this treatment even when family members plead for the order and when the patient's lack of competence to make the decision is evident. See pp. 67–68.

6. In New York, when the condition is life-threatening, ECT may be given with surrogate consent to incapable, non-objecting patients. Surrogate consent is obtained from a family member and the concurrence of the medical director. This consent was challenged in court, but the process was endorsed in 1998 (Disability Advocates et al. vs. J. D. Stone, Supreme Court, New York, July 21, 1998).

7. Parry, 1981; Roy-Byrne and Gerner, 1981. For a layman's description of how California's laws interfered with one patient's treatment see chapter 20 in Wyden, 1988.

8. Since we recognize that the mentally ill may not be able to assess the severity of their illness, we should consider allowing the same leeway in applying electroshock that psychiatrists have in applying psychotropic drugs.

9. The tourniquet is inflated above the systolic blood pressure before the muscle relaxing agent is administered, preventing the agent from affecting the muscles in one limb. The duration of the motor movements of the seizure can then be timed (Fink and Johnson, 1982).

10. The muscle stimulator is a battery-operated device that delivers low-energy pulses to a nerve under the skin, eliciting a twitch in the muscles. Since these may be painful, they are tested after the patient is asleep.

11. The mouth guard is made of rubber or plastic. When the teeth need added protection, an individualized device, similar to that used by athletes in contact sports, is made by a dentist.

12. There is no reason to be concerned that a painful shock or that electrocution will occur. Neither patients nor treatment team members have ever been electrocuted during ECT.

13. Manning, 1994.

14. Endler, 1990.

15. APA, 1990; Fink, 1994; Fink, Abrams, et al., 1996.
16. Fink, 1994, 1995a.
17. The first treatment schedules imitated the frequency of the fevers induced by the malaria treatment of neurosyphilis. See Chapter 10.
18. Fink, 1979; Abrams, 1997a.
19. Maletzky, 1981. An invidious twist in Medicare reimbursement rates allows extra payments to physicians who administer more than one seizure in a treatment. This economic incentive encourages the use of MMECT despite its acknowledged risks and lack of increased efficacy.
20. Murillo and Exner, 1973; Exner and Murillo, 1977. Such treatments relieved severe and unremitting delusional syndromes, especially those dominated by persistent excitement. In its stead, ECT augmentation of antipsychotic drugs is now used.
21. Rich, 1984; Keisling, 1984.
22. Rodger, Scott, and Whalley, 1994.
23. Prien and Kupfer, 1986; Aronson et al., 1987.
24. This practice is similar to that used in pharmacotherapy, where a six-month course is the minimum for the treatment of first episodes, and at least one year of treatment is necessary for a recurrent illness. Lifelong prescription of medications is not unusual for patients with psychosis, mania, or delusional depression.
25. Scientists use rating scales to measure change. The scales consist of individual items that are scored for presence and severity. A change in score to a more normal direction is seen as improvement; a change away from normal is seen as a worsening of the illness. The items usually focus on objective, measurable features of the illness, like appetite, weight, and sleeping patterns. The scale scores support information from family members about the changes in symptoms and the patient's ability to participate in daily life.
26. Prudic et al., 1990; Sackeim et al., 1990.
27. Fink, Abrams, et al., 1996.
28. A group led by Dr. Harold Sackeim at Columbia University, in collaboration with scientists at the University of Pittsburgh and the University of Iowa, addresses continuation treatment with Pamelor alone, Pamelor combined with lithium, or placebo for both medications. A second group, headed by Dr. Charles Kellner at Medical University of South Carolina, in collaboration with scientists at the Long Island Jewish Hillside Medical Center in New York, the University of Texas at Dallas, and the Mayo Clinic in Rochester, Minnesota, studies continuation ECT or continuation with a combination of Pamelor and lithium, the latter in the same schedule as the Sackeim studies. The results of these studies are expected by the year 2001.
29. Petrides et al., 1994; Petrides, in press.

30. Extensive experiences with continuation ECT were described by Moore, 1943; Geoghegan and Stevenson, 1949; Stevenson and Geoghegan, 1951; and Karliner and Wehrheim, 1965. Continuation ECT was not revived when ECT was re-established in the belief that medicines would sustain its benefits, a belief that was encouraged by prevalent ideas that psychotropic drugs and ECT worked by the same mechanisms.
31. Patient Helen Dickinson, Chapter 5.
32. Patient Steven Hancock, Chapter 7.
33. Patients with delusional depression, rapid cycling mania, and paranoid schizophrenia relapse rapidly. Such cases require prolonged treatment.

Chapter 3: Risks and Contraindications

1. Abrams, 1997b.
2. Damascio, 1994.
3. Kiloh, 1961.
4. The patients exhibit a syndrome of confusion, disorientation, excitement, rapid heart rate, and elevated blood pressure, known as anticholinergic delirium. (Fink, 1960; Bradley and Fink, 1968).
5. Abrams, 1997a; Fink, 1979; Sackeim, 1992; Sackeim, Prudic, et al., 1993; Calev, Ben-Tzvi, et al., 1989; Calev, Nigal, et al., 1991; Calev, 1994; Lerer et al., 1995.
6. Janis, 1948, 1950.
7. Holmberg, 1953a, b.
8. Styron, 1990.
9. A Practicing Psychiatrist, 1965.
10. Abrams, 1989, 1997a.
11. Abrams, 1997a; Greenberg, Anand, et al., 1986; Greenberg, Mofson, et al., 1988.
12. Abrams 1989, 1997a.
13. Cizadlo and Wheaton, 1995; Moise and Petrides, 1996; Rey and Walter, 1997; Walter and Rey, 1997; Fink and Coffey, 1998; Ghaziuddin, 1998.

Chapter 4: Technical Features of the Treatment

1. Curare, an effective muscle relaxant, was first used to modify the convulsion in ECT. The duration of curare's effect was often prolonged, inhibiting its use (Bennett 1941, 1972). Succinylcholine was introduced by Holmberg and Thesleff in 1952.
2. Pentothal is another frequently used barbiturate. Amidate and Diprivan are alternatives. For excited patients, Ketalar is a useful agent.

3. A sore throat and a hoarse voice occasionally result from the procedure.

4. An anticholinergic drug also blocks the action of the vagus nerve, the 10th cranial nerve, which arises from the base of the brain. This nerve controls the heart's rate. When an electrical stimulus to the brain does not develop a seizure, as may happen when the energy is too low, or when unilateral electrode placement is selected, the vagus effect will slow the heart and may even stop it momentarily. The anticholinergic drug prevents this effect and keeps the heart beating properly.

5. The sinusoidal form of electrical energy was used widely between 1938 and 1980. It is commonly available from a conventional wall outlet in the United States at 110 volts; in the devices it is reduced to 70 volts or increased to 170 volts by a transformer. A clock, graduated from 0.1 to 1.0 second, controlled a measured amount of energy for the treatment. Such energy is less efficient and is no longer used.

6. The two principal manufacturers of ECT devices in the United States are Somatics Inc. (910 Sherwood Drive, Unit 17, Lake Bluff, IL 60044; 800.642.6761) and the MECTA Corporation (7015 S. W. McEwan Road, Lake Oswego, OR 97035; 503.624.8778).

7. Sackeim, Decina, et al., 1987; Sackeim, Prudic, et al. 1993; Petrides and Fink, 1996b.

8. When an anticipated clinical improvement is not seen after four unilateral treatments, a change to bilateral placement is recommended (Abrams and Fink, 1984).

9. Fink and Johnson, 1982.

10. Abrams, 1997a.

11. Fink and Abrams, 1998.

12. The principal training opportunities in 1999 were at Columbia University (Dr. Harold Sackeim, 212.960.5855), Duke University (Dr. Richard Weiner, 919.681.8742), the Long Island Jewish Hillside Hospital (Dr. Samuel Bailine, 718.470.8025), and the Medical University of South Carolina (Dr. Charles Kellner, 803.792.0053).

    Courses in ECT are also given in conjunction with the annual meetings of the Association for Convulsive Therapy (Dr. Frank Moscarillo, executive secretary, ACT, 301.951.7220). CME Inc. also sponsors ECT training programs (CME Inc., 800. 447.4474).

13. APA, 1990. The specific recommendations are: "Each resident should actively participate in at least 10 ECT treatments directly supervised by a privileged treating psychiatrist, and involving at least three separate cases. Each resident should actively participate in the care of at least two patients during the ECT workup and course of treatments" (p. 43).

14. Fink, Abrams, et al., 1996.

15. In some hospitals, ECT is given in an operating room, although safe treatment does not require it and it is unnecessarily expensive.

Chapter 5: Depressive Mood Disorders

1. APA, 1994.
2. Abrams, 1997a; Coffey, 1993; Kellner, 1991; Fink, 1979.
3. Fink, 1997b.
4. Abrams, 1997a; APA, 1990.
5. Bruce and Leaf, 1989.
6. Rorsman, Hognell, and Lauke, 1986.
7. Singer et al., 1976.
8. Black and Winokur, 1986; Black, Warrack, and Winokur, 1985a.
9. Black, Warrack, and Winokur, 1985b; Black, Wilcox, and Stewart, 1985; Black, Winokur, and Warrack, 1985.
10. Philibert et al., 1995.
11. Avery and Winokur, 1978.
12. APA, 1990.
13. Glassman, Kantor, and Shostak, 1975; Kantor and Glassman, 1977.
14. Kroessler, 1985.
15. Avery and Lubrano, 1979.
16. Kroessler, 1985.
17. Flint and Rifat, 1998.
18. Aronson et al., 1987.
19. Myers, Kalayam, and Mei-Tal, 1984, 1985; Fink, 1986c; Mitchell et al., 1996; Rush et al., 1996; Nelson and Davis, 1997.
20. Mulsant et al., 1997.
21. Abrams, 1998.
22. Chapter 2, note 6.
23. Aronson et al., 1987; Schatzberg and Rothschild, 1993.
24. Coffey, Hinkle, et al., 1987; Coffey, Figiel, et al., 1988a, b; Coffey, Weiner, et al., 1991.
25. Kiloh, 1961.
26. Examples of the stupor and pseudodementia of depression were described as benign stupors. These were often fatal before the introduction of electroshock (Hoch, 1921).
27. Bright-Long and Fink, 1993.
28. Fink, 1997a.
29. Cronkite, 1994.
30. Fink, 1995c; Schneekloth, Rummans, and Logan, 1993; Moise and Petrides, 1996; Rey and Walter, 1997; Walter and Rey, 1997; Cohen et al., 1997.
31. No adjustments to the adult ECT protocol were required except that close attention was given to energy dosing. Adolescents require little

energy to induce an effective seizure. No reporter described instances of uncontrolled seizures.

32. Clardy and Rumpf, 1954; Gurevitz and Helme, 1954; Carr et al., 1983; Black, Wilcox, and Stewart, 1985; Guttmacher and Cretella, 1988; Powell et al., 1988; Cizadlo and Wheaton, 1995.

33. Clardy and Rumpf, 1954.

34. Cizadlo and Wheaton, 1995.

35. Had her condition occurred in another setting, it might well have been erroneously diagnosed as *pervasive refusal syndrome*. A group of British child psychiatrists describe four children "with a potentially life-threatening condition manifested by profound and pervasive refusal to eat, drink, walk, talk, or care for themselves in any way over a period of several months" (Lask et al., 1991). The syndrome is assumed to result from psychological trauma, and the recommended treatment is individual and family psychotherapy. In a report of one such case, an 8-year-old girl suffered a viral infection and some weeks later stopped eating and drinking. She was withdrawn and mute, complained of muscle weakness, developed incontinence of urine and feces, and was unable to walk (Graham and Foreman, 1995). On her admission to a hospital, a diagnosis of pervasive refusal syndrome was made. The child was treated with psychotherapy and family therapy for more than a year, after which she was discharged back to her family.

These cases meet our criteria for catatonia and not depression (Fink, 1997a). The successful use of ECT in the case treated by Cizaldo and Wheaton was lauded, and the failure to treat the second case for catatonia, either with ECT or with benzodiazepines, was criticized (Fink and Klein, 1995). The significance of the distinction in therapists' attitudes toward catatonia and pervasive refusal syndrome is in the treatment options available to the patient. If the pervasive refusal syndrome is viewed as the result of psychological trauma, to be treated by individual and family psychotherapy, then a slow and limited recovery described in the second patient may result. If the syndrome is viewed as an example of catatonia, however, then the options of sedative drugs (Amytal, Valium, Ativan) are available, and when these fail, recourse to electroshock has a good prognosis.

36. Thuppal and Fink, in press.

37. The Texas legislature had already banned ECT for anyone under the age of 16.

38. Examples of the experiences of mentally ill authors during ECT are found in Freeman, 1986; Gotkin and Gotkin, 1975; Plath, 1971; Steir, 1978; and Vonnegut, 1975.

39. Flach, 1990: Chapters 30–32, pp. 130–39, and the epilogue, p. 271.

Chapter 6: Manic Mood Disorders

1. Bond, 1980; Fink, in press.
2. Rapid neuroleptization called for repeated intravenous doses of Haldol to induce a speedy response. The procedure carries a high risk of death and neuroleptic malignant syndrome. It is generally discarded now.
3. A review of the reports of manic patients treated with electroshock found 371 of 562 (66 percent) remitted or showed marked clinical improvement (Mukherjee, Sackeim, and Schnur, 1994).
4. Miller, 1995. See also pp. 67–68.
5. Murillo and Exner, 1973; Exner and Murillo, 1977.
6. Meduna, 1937; Fink and Sackeim, 1996.
7. Recent studies find a more effective combination in the use of Clozaril combined with ECT (Klapheke, 1989; Landy, 1991; Safferman and Munne, 1992; Green et al., 1994; Fink, 1998).
8. Abrams and Taylor, 1976; Taylor and Abrams, 1973, 1977; Bräunig et al., 1998.

Chapter 7: Thought Disorders

1. Fink, 1995b.
2. Fink, Shaw et al., 1958.
3. Kane and Smith, 1982; Kane, Woerner, et al., 1984; Woerner et al., 1998.
4. As more experience with these drugs develops, descriptions of toxic conditions, including the neuroleptic malignant syndrome, are emerging (Hasan and Buckley, 1998).
5. Kane, Honigfeld, et al., 1988.
6. Most new psychotropic medicines come to the market with limited testing, mainly in moderately ill adults for short periods. Understanding of the true efficacy and risks comes in the clinic, among patients who are treated without being told that the effects of the compounds are poorly known. Experience with electroshock is far more extensive, and the family of a psychotic patient who is responding poorly to psychotropic drugs should ask what experience the psychiatrist has had with the prescribed medicines, and whether he or she has considered electroshock as an alternative.
7. Klapheke, 1989; Fink and Sackeim, 1996
8. Aird and Strait, 1945; Bolwig, Hertz, Holm-Jensen, et al., 1977; Bolwig, Hertz, Paulson, et al., 1977.
9. Fink, 1998.
10. Christison et al., 1991; Wyatt, 1991.
11. Sadly, the algorithms for treatment of psychosis developed by expert committees do not consider the role of electroshock until many drug trials are done, including trials of new psychotropic medicines (APA,

1997; McEvoy et al., 1996). The same neglect is seen in reviews of treatment options for schizophrenia (Kane and McGlashan, 1995). A change, however, may be evident in the Texas Medication Algorithm Project which includes electroshock after two medication trials have failed (Gilbert et al., 1998; Crismon et al., 1999).

12. Fink and Kahn, 1957.
13. Flumazenil is a rapidly active brain receptor antagonist to the action of benzodiazepines. It makes possible the option of ECT for patients who have taken large doses of benzodiazepines for long periods (Bailine et al., 1994).
14. Wyden, 1998.
15. He reports that reading Berton Roueché's 1974 article in *The New Yorker* magazine was most discouraging.
16. Wyden 1998, pp. 215–16.
17. The doctor's failure to prescribe an adequate course of continuation ECT prolonged Jeff's illness and caused the father to believe, erroneously, that ECT had failed his son. Jeff eventually responded to a new atypical neuroleptic medication, Zyprexa, and was discharged to the community. A review for Peter Wyden's book stated that it *"outlines a new treatment that many consider the safest, most effective to date"* (*New York Times Book Review*, June 21, 1998, p. 3).

Chapter 8: Movement Disorders

1. Kahlbaum, 1973.
2. McCall et al., 1995.
3. Abrams and Taylor, 1976; Abrams et al., 1979; Gelenberg 1976; Gelenberg and Mandel, 1977; Taylor and Abrams, 1973, 1977; Taylor, 1990; Fink, 1997a.
4. Fink and Taylor, 1991. Rating scales help caregivers to recognize the syndrome (Bush et al., 1996a; Bräunig et al., 1998).
5. APA, 1994. This classification recognizes the class 293.89 of "catatonic disorder due to . . . (indicate the general medical condition)."
6. Taylor, 1990; Fink and Taylor, 1991; Bush et al., 1996a, b.
7. Fink, 1996a.
8. Fink, 1996a.
9. Lazarus, Mann, and Caroff, 1989.
10. Fink, 1996a.
11. Fink, 1996b.
12. Lebensohn and Jenkins, 1975.
13. Balldin, Eden et al., 1980; Balldin, Granerus, et al., 1981; Andersen et al., 1987.
14. Douyon et al., 1989; Zervas and Fink, 1991; Rasmussen and Abrams, 1991; Faber and Trimble, 1991.

15. Zervas and Fink, 1991; Figiel et al., 1991; Faber, 1992; Fink and Zervas, 1992.
16. Fink, 1995b.
17. Working Group, 1993.
18. Lowenstein and Alldredge, 1998.
19. Caplan (1945, 1946). Recent case reports re-enforce the usefulness of this procedure (Sackeim et al., 1983; Schnur et al., 1989; Viparelli and Viparelli, 1992; Griesemer et al., 1997).
20. Abrams, 1997.
21. Trimble, 1978; Fenton, 1986.
22. Bye, Nunn, and Wilson, 1985; Tomson et al., 1989. One explanation for the failure to release prolactin is that the pituitary stores are exhausted. This suggestion is contradicted, however, by two elegant studies that found that prolactin is still released by thyrotropin-releasing hormone or metoclopramide in patients in SE (Lindblom et al., 1992, 1993).
23. Fink, Kellner, and Sackeim, in press. In the event that an effective seizure is not induced in a patient who has recently been given large doses of benzodiazepines, their activity can be blocked by graduated doses of the antagonist flumazenil before introducing an ECT seizure (Bailine et al., 1994; Krystal et al., 1998).

Chapter 9: How Does It Work?

1. Many theories have been developed, each focused on a single aspect of the treatment that was of interest at the time. In 1958, encouraged by psychodynamic beliefs, I followed the writings of Weinstein and Kahn (1955) in formulating a physiologic-dynamic view of ECT (Fink, 1957). When this was no longer satisfactory, I studied acetylcholine as a messenger substance in the brain and formulated a cholinergic hypothesis (Fink, 1966). This hypothesis was also discarded. The neuroendocrine discoveries soon seemed more cogent, and I developed the neuroendocrine view (Fink, 1979, 1990). This view seems to me to be the most cogent explanation of ECT within our understanding of brain function, behavior, mental illness, and seizures.
2. Fink, 1979, pp. 24–26.
3. Usdin, Hamburg, and Barchas, 1977; Nemeroff and Loosen, 1987.
4. Berson and Yalow, 1968.
5. Many researchers thought that direct stimulation of the hypothalamus was essential and that the production of a seizure was not necessary for the behavioral outcome. Electrical stimulation of the brain through midline electrodes, with one needle in the upper lip and the second in the vertex of the scalp, in electro-acupuncture ECT elicited the same effects as bitemporal electrode placement, but only when

grand mal seizures were elicited (Dingxiong and Zhuosu, 1985; Chongcheng et al., 1985). Direct hypothalamic stimulation is an aim of studies in rapid transcranial stimulation (rTMS).

6. The burden for rTMS, a proposed replacement for electroshock, is to demonstrate changes in neuroendocrine regulation and products in conjunction with persistent clinical benefits.

7. Berson and Yalow, 1968. Dr. Yalow's report of the measurement of the release of ACTH in ECT led to her 1977 Nobel Prize for Physiology and Medicine (Straus, 1998).

8. Bergland, 1985.

9. The most promising candidate has been thyrotropin-releasing-hormone (TRH), a tripeptide released by the hypothalamus. It has euphoriant and antidepressant effects when given parenterally to humans. Because it is rapidly metabolized, however, its action is short. A congener of TRH with robust resistance to metabolic denigration is a reasonable target of chemical research. Such congeners to other brain peptides, for beta-endorphin, des-Tyr-γ-endorphin (GK-78, Organon), and for vasopressin, desglycinamide ariginine vasopressin (Org 5667, Organon), are examples of modified brain peptides with longer durations of action than the natural compounds.

10. The hormonal explanation is criticized as either unproved and too vague to be testable (Sackeim and Devanand, 1990) and as superseded by a theory of kindling (Post, 1990). The thyroid gland and its response to the pituitary is seen as a more likely candidate for the antidepressant effects of electroshock (Nutt, 1990). The most common criticism is that the neuroendocrine theory ignores our knowledge of the brain's neurohumors, whose actions are the most common explanation of the efficacy of psychotropic drugs (Cooper, Scott, and Whalley, 1990; Sackeim, 1989). An example of such thinking is that of King and Liston (1990), who visualize convulsive therapy as a nonspecific, nonphysiologic depolarization of neurons which then allows the brain's diseased ratios of brain neurotransmitters to become normal.

11. Nemeroff and Loosen, 1987, Nemeroff, Bissette, et al., 1991.

Chapter 10: The Origins of Electroshock Therapy

1. Klaesi, 1922.

2. Grob, 1985 (pp. 109–16).

3. Adolf Meyer, professor of psychiatry at Johns Hopkins Hospital, was an active supporter of the eugenics movement.

4. Grob, 1985 (p. 171); Grob, 1994 (pp. 160–61).

5. Schönbauer and Jantsch, 1950; Terry, 1939.

6. Wagner-Jauregg, 1918.

7. Alternative sources of fevers are: relapsing fever instead of malaria; injections of gonococcal vaccine; typhoid vaccine; tuberculin; or milk, to induce protein sensitivity fevers; and elevations of body core temperatures by electric blankets and enclosed cabinets heated by electric lights. These methods were no more successful than malarial fevers.

8. Dattner, 1944; Duffy, 1995.

9. The belief in the release of substances into the blood that could be therapeutic was a feature of Ugo Cerletti's explanation for the efficacy of electroshock (Cerletti, 1950). He named the substances *acroagonines* and looked for them in the cerebrospinal fluid. His experiments called for spinal fluid to be transferred from epileptic patients to those with dementia praecox.

10. Meduna, 1985.

11. Meduna, 1935.

12. Meduna, 1935.

13. Meduna, 1985.

14. Meduna, 1937.

15. Katzenelbogen and Santee, 1938. Much of the proceedings were devoted to studies of insulin coma.

16. For his autobiography, see Meduna, 1985. Meduna's contribution in creating a new and effective treatment is well documented. In the United States he developed another novel treatment, carbon dioxide therapy, an attempt to alter brain function by physiologic means. This method was unsuccessful (Meduna, 1950a). He also described the psychopathology of manic delirium in an essay called *Oneirophrenia* (1950b). He was aided in his admission to the United States by Dr. Victor Gonda, a Hungarian neuropsychiatrist.

17. Weigert, 1940.

18. Cerletti, 1950, 1956; Bini, 1938.

19. Cerletti, 1956, p. 93; Bini, 1995.

20. By 1940, reports appeared of the Metrazol treatment of 3,000 cases in the United States and 2,011 in Europe (Jessner and Ryan, 1941).

21. Abrams, 1988.

22. The cavalier and adventurous attitudes of physicians were not limited to those who sought to develop somatic therapies for mental illness. The same attitudes encouraged psychotherapists, whose results were just as untested and just as disastrous to their patients (Shorter, 1997; Braslow, 1998; Dolnick, 1998).

23. For a description of the enthusiasm with which fever therapy was accepted, despite its risks and poor results, see Duffy, 1995.

24. Legislative actions in various states, especially California, led the American Psychiatric Association to organize a Task Force on Electroconvulsive Therapy under the chairmanship of Dr. Fred Frankel

of Boston. After finding that the efficacy of ECT warranted its continued use, the members proposed a formal consent process to reduce
the likelihood that ECT would be used in non-consenting patients.
The consent guidelines have been widely adopted in psychiatric practice, and endorsed by a second Task Force in 1990, which reviewed
the interim experience. (American Psychiatric Association, 1978,
1990).

Chapter 11: Controversy in Electroshock

1. Deutsch, 1937, 1948.
2. Beers, 1908.
3. Frankel, 1973; Grosser et al., 1975.
4. Spock, 1946, 1957, 1968, 1976, 1985, 1992.
5. In a well-publicized case, Dr. Osheroff, a hospitalized depressed patient, was treated with intensive psychotherapy without benefit. He
   recovered with psychotropic drugs in another hospital. His lawsuit
   over the doctors' failure to follow through with biological treatment
   for the proper diagnosis of depression was settled in his favor (Klerman, 1990).
6. Group for the Advancement of Psychiatry, 1947. The report was issued from the Menninger Foundation in Topeka, Kansas.
7. D'Agostino, 1975; Lebensohn, 1984; Fink, 1984, 1991, 1997d.
8. Fink, 1997d.
9. A sad example is the life of Philip Graham, the publisher of the
   Washington Post and *Newsweek* and an influential figure in the
   Washington political scene for almost two decades. His six-year
   struggle with manic-depressive illness was treated with psychotherapy, then with medications. He committed suicide. The highs and
   lows of the illness are clearly described by his wife, Katherine Graham, in a memorable autobiography (Graham, 1997a), and even more
   poignantly in readings available on audiotape (Graham, 1997b).
10. Three proper studies of Thorazine and insulin coma found Thorazine
    to be as effective as insulin coma, less expensive to administer, and
    safer (Ackner et al., 1957; Boardman et al., 1956; Fink, Shaw, et al.,
    1958). By 1960 the insulin coma units in the United States were
    closed.
11. For a review of the various evaluations of ECT, see Fink, 1991. The
    major reports are those of the American Psychiatric Association in
    1978 and 1990, the Royal College of Psychiatrists (Pippard and Ellam,
    1981), and the Irish Royal College of Psychiatrists (Latey and Fahy,
    1982). A major review was undertaken by the National Institute of
    Mental Health in the Consensus Conference, 1985. The studies that
    summarize the efficacy of ECT in various mental states are detailed

in major textbooks such as Fink (1979) and Abrams (1997a). Many
of the individual reports are cited in the clinical sections in this book.

12. Frankel, 1973; Grosser et al., 1975.
13. Kramer, 1985; in press.
14. Reid et al., 1998.
15. Kramer, 1985; in press.
16. Szasz, 1960.
17. Breggin 1979, 1991.
18. Isaac and Armat, 1990.
19. Anonymous, 1992; Röder, Kubillus, and Burwell, 1995.
20. Cauchon, 1995; Solomon, 1998; Stone, 1994.
21. Cauchon, 1995.
22. APA, 1978.
23. Pippard and Ellam, 1981.
24. Editor, 1981.
25. Pippard, 1992.
26. Duffett and Lelliott, 1997, 1998; Trezise, 1998.
27. Latey and Fahy, 1982.
28. Clark, 1985.
29. Consensus Conference, 1985.
30. AMA, 1989.
31. News & Notes, 1992, 1993, 9: 69–73.
32. Squire, 1987.
33. Stone, 1994.
34. Fink, Kety et al., 1974.
35. Malitz and Sackeim, 1986.
36. APA, 1990. In 1997, the APA authorized a third assessment, due in
    1999.
37. Consensus Conference, 1992.
38. Hermann, Ettner, et al., 1998.
39. The family of a patient referred for ECT should certainly inquire as
    to the training and experience of the practitioner who will provide
    the treatment. The necessary skills to assure safe and effective treat-
    ments are not widely distributed among physicians.
40. The need for certifying examinations and continuing medical edu-
    cation standards in this evolving discipline are under consideration
    by the members of the Association for Convulsive Therapy.
41. Duffett and Lelliott, 1997, 1998.

Chapter 12: Electroshock in the 1990s

1. Hermann, Dowart, et al., 1995.
2. Thompson et al., 1994.
3. See case of Jeffrey Cooper, Chapter 8.

4. APA, 1978.
5. Sackeim, Prudic, et al., 1993.
6. The new devices also enable practitioners to monitor the seizure EEG, electromyogram (for motor duration of the seizure), and the electro-cardiogram (for an estimate of duration by heart rate).
7. Fink and Johnson, 1982.
8. Kellner and Fink, 1996; Fink and Abrams, 1998.
9. Fink and Kahn, 1957.
10. Abrams, Fink, et al., 1972; Abrams, Volavka, et al., 1973; Sackeim, Luber, et al., 1996. Also, Kellner and Fink, 1996.
11. None of these presentations includes consideration of electroshock even in regard to illnesses in which efficacy is not questioned, as in the treatment of therapy-resistant depression, mania, or acute psychoses.
12. 100 Joules (504 millicoulombs) at 220 ohms impedance.
13. Sackeim, 1991; Abrams 1997a.
14. For some elderly patients, psychiatrists must now use cumbersome and riskier techniques, such as the administration of caffeine or theophylline (Nobler and Sackeim, 1993) or double stimulation (Swartz and Mehta, 1986; Andrade, 1991). The double-stimulation method has been criticized (Swartz, 1991). Most egregious is the unnecessary increased numbers of treatments and treatment failures as a consequence of federal regulations that make useful equipment unavailable in the United States.
15. Higher-energy devices are available for research purposes at the principal academic research centers in the country. They have been used safely and effectively for more than a decade.
16. Fink and Bailine, 1998; Bailine, 1998.
17. Markowitz et al., 1987.
18. Steffens et al., 1995.
19. Olfson et al., 1998.
20. Rodger, Scott, and Whalley, 1994.
21. Insurers are dependent on treatment algorithms proposed by academic committees. Such treatment algorithms are published as supplements to the *American Journal of Psychiatry* and other journals, and become established as guidelines for treatment. Unfortunately, the algorithms either fail to consider electroshock or cite it only as a last resort, thereby giving weight to inappropriate treatment schedules as national standards.
22. The first algorithms to include electroshock have just been published from the Texas Medication Algorithm Project (Crismon et al., 1999).

Bibliography

Abrams R. Interview with Lothar Kalinowsky, M.D. *Convulsive Ther* 1988; 4: 24–39.

Abrams R (ed). ECT in the high-risk patient. *Convulsive Ther* 1989; 5: 1–118.

Abrams R. *Electroconvulsive Therapy*. Third ed., 382 pp. Oxford Univ Press, New York, 1997a.

Abrams R. The mortality rate with ECT. *Convulsive Ther* 1997b; 13: 125–7.

Abrams R. ECT and psychotic depression, *Am J Psychiatry* 1998; 155: 306–7.

Abrams R, Fink M. The present status of unilateral ECT: Some recommendations. *J Affect Disord* 1984; 7: 245–7.

Abrams R, Fink M, Dornbush R, et al. Unilateral and bilateral ECT: Effects on depression, memory and the electroencephalogram. *Arch Gen Psychiatry* 1972; 27: 88–94.

Abrams R, Swartz C. *What You Need to Know About Electroconvulsive Therapy*. Information booklet. Somatics Inc., 1991.

Abrams R, Taylor M A. Catatonia, a prospective clinical study. *Arch Gen Psychiatry* 1976; 33: 579–81.

Abrams R, Taylor M A, Stolurow K A: Catatonia and mania: Patterns of cerebral dysfunction. *Biol Psychiatry* 1979; 14: 111–17.

Abrams R, Volavka J, Fink M. EEG seizure patterns during multiple unilateral and bilateral ECT. *Comprehens Psychiatry* 1973; 14: 25–8.

Ackner B, Harris A, Oldham A J. Insulin treatment of schizophrenia. Controlled study. *Lancet* 1957; 2: 607–11.

Aird R B, Strait I. Protective barriers of the central nervous system: An experimental study with trypan red. *Arch Neurol Psychiatry* 1945; 51: 54–66.

American Medical Association. AMA supports use of ECT. *Convulsive Ther* 1989; 5: 199.

American Psychiatric Association. *Electroconvulsive Therapy*. 200 pp. Washington, D.C., 1978.

American Psychiatric Association. *Electroconvulsive Therapy: Recommendations for Treatment, Training and Privileging*. 186 pp. Washington, D.C., 1990.

American Psychiatric Association. *Diagnostic and Statistical Manual of Mental Disorders.* Fourth ed., 886 pp. Washington, D.C., 1994.

American Psychiatric Association. Practice guidelines for the treatment of patients with schizophrenia. *Am J Psychiatry* 1997; 154: Supplement 1–63.

Andersen K, Balldin J, Gottfries C G, et al. A double-blind evaluation of electroconvulsive therapy in Parkinson's disease with "on-off" phenomena. *Acta Neurol Scand* 1987; 76: 191–9.

Andrade C. Double stimulation to elicit an adequate treatment. *Convulsive Ther* 1991; 300–1.

Anonymous. *What Is Scientology?* 833 pp. Bridge Publications, Los Angeles, 1992.

Aronson T, Shukla S, Hoff A. Continuation therapy after ECT for delusional depression. A naturalistic study of prophylactic treatments and relapse. *Convulsive Ther* 1987; 3: 251–9.

Avery D, Lubrano A. Depression treated with imipramine and ECT: The deCarolis study reconsidered. *Am J Psychiatry* 1979; 136: 559–62

Avery D, Winokur G. Suicide, attempted suicide, and relapse rates in depression. *Arch Gen Psychiatry* 1978; 35: 749–53.

Bailine S. Reimbursement and documentation issues in an ambulatory ECT program. *JECT*, 1998; 14: 255–8.

Bailine S H, Safferman A, Vital-Herne J, et al. Flumazenil reversal of benzodiazepine-induced sedation for a patient with severe pre-ECT anxiety. *Convulsive Ther* 1994, 10: 65–8.

Balldin J, Eden S, Granerus A K, et al. Electroconvulsive therapy in Parkinson's syndrome with "on-off" phenomenon. *J Neural Transm* 1980; 47: 11–21.

Balldin J, Granerus A K, Lindstedt G, et al. Predictors for improvement after electroconvulsive therapy in Parkinsonian patients with on-off symptoms. *J Neural Transm* 1981; 52: 199–211.

Beers C. *A Mind That Found Itself.* Longmans, Green & Co, New York, 1908.

Bennett A E. Curare. A preventive of traumatic complications in convulsive shock therapy. Including a report on a synthetic curare-like drug. *Am J Psychiatry* 1941; 97: 1040–60.

Bennett A E. *Fifty Years in Neurology and Psychiatry.* 166 pp. Intercontinental Book Publishing Co., New York, 1972.

Bergland R. *The Fabric of Mind.* 202 pp. Penguin Books, Middlesex, England, 1985.

Berson S, Yalow R. Radioimmunoassay of ACTH in plasma. *J Clin Invest* 1968; 47: 2725–51.

Bini L. Experimental researches on epileptic attacks induced by the electric current. In Katzenelbogen S, Santee F. *The Treatment of Schizophre-*

nia: *Insulin Shock, Cardiozol, Sleep Treatment. Am J Psychiatry* 1938; 94: Supplement 172–4.

Bini L. Professor Bini's notes on the first electro-shock experiment. *Convulsive Ther* 1995; 11: 260–1.

Black D W, Warrack G, Winokur G. Excess mortality among psychiatric patients: The Iowa record-linkage study. *Journal of American Medical Association* 1985a; 253: 58–61.

Black D W, Warrack G, Winokur G. I: Suicides and accidental deaths among psychiatric patients: The Iowa record-linkage study. *Arch Gen Psychiatry* 1985b; 42: 71–5.

Black D W, Warrack G, Winokur G. II: Excess mortality among patients with organic mental disorders: The Iowa record-linkage study. *Arch Gen Psychiatry* 1985c; 42: 78–81.

Black D W, Wilcox J A, Stewart M. The use of ECT in children: Case report. *J Clin Psychiatry* 1985; 46: 98–9.

Black D W, Winokur G. Prospective studies of suicide and mortality in psychiatric patients. *Annals NY Acad Sci* 1986; 487: 106–13.

Black D W, Winokur G, Warrack G. Suicide in schizophrenia: The Iowa record-linkage study. *J Clin Psychiatry* 1985; 46: 14–17.

Boardman R H, Lomas J, Markowe M. Insulin and chlorpromazine in schizophrenia: Comparative study of previously untreated cases. *Lancet* 1956; 2: 487–94.

Bolwig T, Hertz M M, Holm-Jensen J. Blood-brain barrier permeability during electroshock seizures in the rat. *Eur J Clin Invest* 1977; 7: 95–100.

Bolwig T, Hertz M M, Paulson O B, et al. The permeability of the blood-brain barrier during electrically induced seizures in man. *Eur J Clin Invest* 1977; 7: 87–93.

Bond T C. Recognition of acute delirious mania. *Arch Gen Psychiatry* 1980; 37: 553–4.

Bourne H. Insulin myth. *Lancet* 1953; 2: 964–8.

Bradley P, Fink M (eds). *Anticholinergic Drugs and Brain Functions in Animals and Man. Progress in Brain Research* 28: 184 pp. Elsevier, Amsterdam. 1968.

Braslow J. *Mental Illness and Bodily Cures.* University of California Press, Berkeley, 1998.

Bräunig P, Krüger S, Shugar G. Prevalence and clinical significance of catatonic symptoms in mania. *Comprehens Psychiatry* 1998; 39: 35–46.

Breggin P R. *Electro-Shock. Its Brain-Disabling Effects.* 244 pp. Springer, New York, 1979.

Breggin P R. *Toxic Psychiatry: Why Therapy, Empathy, and Love Must Replace the Drugs, Electroshock, and Biochemical Theories of the "New Psychiatry."* 464 pp. St. Martin's Press, New York. 1991.

Bright-Long L, Fink M. Reversible dementia and affective disorder: The Rip van Winkle syndrome. *Convulsive Ther* 1993; 9: 209–16.

Bruce M L, Leaf P J. Psychiatric disorders and 15-month mortality in a community sample of older adults. *Am J Public Hlth* 1989; 79: 727–30.

Bush G, Fink M, Petrides G, et al. Catatonia: I: Rating scale and standardized examination. *Acta Psychiatr Scand* 1996a; 93: 129–36.

Bush G, Fink M, Petrides G, et al. Catatonia: II. Treatment with lorazepam and electroconvulsive therapy. *Acta Psychiatr Scand* 1996b; 93: 137–43.

Bye A M, Nunn K P, Wilson J. Prolactin and seizure activity. *Arch Dis Childhood* 1985; 60: 848–51.

Calev A. Neuropsychology and ECT: Past and future research trends. *Psychopharmacol Bull* 1994; 30: 461–9.

Calev A, Ben-Tzvi E, Shapira B., et al. Distinct memory impairments following electroconvulsive therapy and imipramine. *Psycholog Med* 1989; 19: 111–9.

Calev A, Nigal D, Shapira B, et al. Early and long-term effects of electroconvulsive therapy and depression on memory and other cognitive functions. *J Nerv Ment Dis* 1991; 179: 526–33.

Caplan G. Electrical convulsion therapy in treatment of epilepsy. *J Ment Sci* 1946; 784–93.

Caplan G. Treatment of epilepsy by electrically induced convulsions. A preliminary report. *BMJ* 1945; 1: 511–12.

Carr V, Dorrington C, Schrader G, et al. The use of ECT for mania in childhood bipolar disorder. *Br J Psychiatry* 1983; 143: 411–5.

Cauchon D. Electroshock: Controversy and questions. *USA Today*, Dec. 6–9, 1995.

Cerletti U. Old and new information about electroshock. *Am J Psychiatry* 1950; 107: 87–94.

Cerletti U. Electroshock therapy. In F Marti-Ibanez, R R Sackler, A M Sackler, M D Sackler (eds.) *The Great Physiodynamic Therapies in Psychiatry: An Historical Reappraisal*, pp. 91–120. Hoeber-Harper, New York, 1956.

Chongcheng X, Huansen X, Qingchi R, et al. Electric acupuncture convulsive therapy. *Convulsive Ther* 1985; 1:243–51.

Christison G W, Kirch D G, Wyatt R J. When symptoms persist: Choosing among alternative treatments for schizophrenia. *Schizophrenia Bull* 1991; 17: 217–45.

Cizadlo B C, Wheaton A. ECT Treatment of a young girl with catatonia: A case study. *J Am Acad Child Adol Psychiatry* 1995; 34: 332–5.

Clardy E R, Rumpf E M. The effect of electric shock on children having schizophrenic manifestations. *Psychiatric Q.* 1954; 28: 616–23.

Clark C J. *Report of the Electro-Convulsive Therapy Review Committee,* pp. 95–7. Ontario Government Bookstore, Toronto, 1985.

Coffey C E (ed). *The Clinical Science of Electroconvulsive Therapy.* 259 pp. APA Press, Washington, D.C. 1993.

Coffey C E, Figiel G S, Djang W T, et al. Leukoencephalopathy in elderly depressed patients referred for ECT. *Biol Psychiatry* 1988a; 24: 143–61.

Coffey C E, Figiel G S, Djang W T, et al. Effects of ECT on brain structure: A pilot prospective magnetic resonance imaging study. *Am J Psychiatry* 1988b; 145: 701–6.

Coffey C E, Hinkle P E, Weiner R D, et al. Electroconvulsive therapy of depression in patients with white matter hyperintensity. *Biol Psychiatry* 1987; 22: 629–36.

Coffey C E, Weiner R D, Djang W T, et al. Brain anatomic effects of electroconvulsive therapy: A prospective magnetic resonance imaging study. *Arch Gen Psychiatry* 1991; 48: 1013–21.

Cohen D, Cottias C, Basquin M. Cotard's syndrome in a 15-year-old girl. *Acta Psychiatr Scand* 1997; 95: 164–5.

Consensus Conference. Electroconvulsive therapy. *Journal of American Medical Association* 1985; 254: 103–8.

Consensus Conference. Diagnosis and treatment of depression in late life. *Journal of American Medical Association* 1992; 268: 1018–24.

Cooper S J, Scott A I F, Whalley L J. A neuroendocrine view of ECT. *Br J Psychiatry* 1990; 157: 740–3.

Crismon M L, Trivedi M, Pigott T A et al. The Texas Medication Algorithm Project: Report of the Texas consensus conference panel on medication treatment of major depressive disorder. *J Clin Psychiatry* 1999; 60: 142–56.

Cronkite K. *On the Edge of Darkness; Conversations About Conquering Depression,* pp. 282–91. Doubleday, New York, 1994.

D'Agostino A. Depression: Schism in contemporary psychiatry. *Am J Psychiatry* 1975; 132: 629–32.

Damascio A R. *Descartes' Error: Emotion, Reason and the Human Brain.* 312 pp. G. P. Putnam's Sons, New York, 1994.

Dattner B. *The Management of Neurosyphilis.* 398 pp. Grune & Stratton, New York, 1944.

Deutsch A. *The Mentally Ill in America.* Doubleday, Doran & Co., New York, 1937.

Deutsch A. *The Shame of the States.* Harcourt Brace & Co., New York, 1948.

Dingxiong H, Zhuosun L. Electroconvulsive therapy and electroacupuncture convulsive therapy in China. *Convulsive Ther* 1985; 1: 234–41.

Dolnick E. *Madness on the Couch: Blaming the Victim in the Heyday of Psychoanalysis.* Simon & Schuster, New York, 1998.

Douyon R, Serby M, Klutchko B, et al. ECT and Parkinson's disease revisited: A naturalistic study. *Am J Psychiatry* 1989; 146: 1451–5.

Duffett R, Lelliott P. Junior doctors' training in the theory and the practice of electroconvulsive therapy. *Psychiatric Bull* 1997; 21: 563–5.

Duffett R, Lelliott P. Auditing electroconvulsive therapy. The third cycle. *Br J Psychiatry* 1998; 172: 401–5.

Duffy J D. General paralysis of the insane: Neuropsychiatry's first challenge. *J Neuropsychiatry* 1995; 7: 243–9.

Editor. ECT in Britain: A shameful state of affairs. *The Lancet* 1981; 1: 1207–8.

Endler N. *Holiday of Darkness. A Psychologist's Personal Journey Out of His Depression.* John Wiley & Sons, New York, 1982.

Exner J E, Murillo L G. A long-term follow-up of schizophrenics treated with regressive ECT. *Dis Nerv Syst* 1977; 38: 162–8.

Faber R. More on ECT and delirium in Parkinson's disease. Letter. *J Neuropsychiatry Clin Neurosci* 1992; 4: 232.

Faber R, Trimble M R. Electroconvulsive therapy in Parkinson's disease and other movement disorders. *Movement Disord* 1991; 6: 293–303.

Fenton G W. Epilepsy and hysteria. *Br J Psychiatry* 1986; 149: 28–37.

Figiel G S, Hassen M A, Zorumski C, et al. ECT-induced delirium in depressed patients with Parkinson's disease. *J Neuropsychiatry Clin Neurosci* 1991; 3: 405–11.

Fink M. A unified theory of the action of physiodynamic therapies. *J Hillside Hosp* 1957; 6: 197–206.

Fink M. Effects of anticholinergic compounds on post-convulsive EEG and behavior of psychiatric patients. *EEG Clin Neurophysiol* 1960; 12: 359–69.

Fink M. Cholinergic aspects of convulsive therapy. *J Nerv Ment Dis* 1966; 142: 475–84.

Fink M. *Convulsive Therapy: Theory and Practice.* 308 pp. Raven Press, New York, 1979.

Fink M. Meduna and the origins of convulsive therapy. *Am J Psychiatry* 1984; 141: 1034–41.

Fink M. *Informed ECT for Health Professionals.* Informational videotape. Somatics Inc., Lake Bluff, IL, 1986a.

Fink M. *Informed ECT for Patients and Families.* Informational videotape. Somatics Inc., Lake Bluff, IL, 1986b.

Fink M. Neuroendocrine predictors of electroconvulsive therapy outcome: Dexamethasone suppression tests and prolactin. *Ann NY Acad Sci* 1986c; 462: 30–6.

Fink M. ECT for Parkinson's disease? *Convulsive Ther* 1988; 4: 189–91.

Fink M. How does convulsive therapy work? *Neuropsychopharmacology* 1990; 3: 73–82.

Fink M. Impact of the anti-psychiatry movement on the revival of ECT in the U.S. *Psychiatric Clinics N.A.* 1991; 14: 793–801.

Fink M. Convalescence and ECT. *Convulsive Ther* 1994; 10: 301–3.

Fink M. Convalescence and ECT. Comment on letter by Dr. Brackin. *Convulsive Ther* 1995a; 11: 220–1.

Fink M. Convulsive therapy in delusional disorders. *Psych Clin North America* 1995b; 18: 393–406.

Fink M. Reconsidering ECT in adolescents. *Psych Times* 1995c; 12: 18–19.

Fink M. Neuroleptic malignant syndrome and catatonia: One entity or two? *Biol Psychiatry* 1996a; 39: 1–4.

Fink M. Toxic serotonin syndrome or neuroleptic malignant syndrome? Case report. *Pharmacopsychiatry* 1996b; 29: 159–61.

Fink M. Catatonia. In M Trimble and J Cummings (eds). *Contemporary Behavioural Neurology* 1997a; Chapter 16 pp. 289–309. Butterworth/Heinemann, Oxford, UK.

Fink, M. The decision to use ECT: For whom? When? In A J Rush (ed), *Mood Disorders: Systematic Medication Management. Modern Problems Pharmacopsychiatry* 1997b, pp. 203–14. Karger, Basel, Switzerland.

Fink M. Energy dosing in ECT: Threshold stimulation or formula? *Convulsive Ther* 1997c; 13: 4–6.

Fink, M. Prejudice against ECT: Competition with psychological philosophies as a contribution to its stigma. *Convulsive Ther* 1997d; 13: 253–65.

Fink M. ECT and clozapine in schizophrenia (editorial) *JECT*, 1998; 14: 223–6.

Fink M. Delirious mania. *Bipolar Disorders* (in press).

Fink M, Abrams R. EEG monitoring in ECT: A guide to treatment efficacy. *Psych Times* 1998; 15: 70–2.

Fink M, Abrams R, Bailine S, Jaffe R. Ambulatory electroconvulsive therapy. Task Force Report #1 of the Association for Convulsive Therapy. *Convulsive Ther* 1996; 12: 42–55.

Fink M, Bailine S. Electroconvulsive therapy and managed care. *Am Jrl Managed Care.* 1998; 4: 107–12.

Fink M, Coffey C E. Electroconvulsive therapy in pediatric neuropsychiatry. In C E Coffey and R A Brumback (eds), *Textbook of Pediatric Neuropsychiatry*, pp. 1389–1408. American Psychiatric Press, Washington, D.C. 1998.

Fink M, Johnson L. Monitoring the duration of electroconvulsive therapy seizures: "Cuff" and EEG methods compared. *Arch Gen Psychiatry* 1982; 39: 1189–91.

Fink M, Kahn R L. Relation of EEG delta activity to behavioral response in electroshock: Quantitative serial studies. *Arch Neurol Psychiatry* 1957; 78: 516–25.

Fink M, Kellner C H, Sackeim H A. Intractable seizures, status epilepticus, and ECT. *JECT* (in press).

Fink M, Kety S, McGaugh J. *Psychobiology of Convulsive Therapy.* 312 pp. V H Winston & Sons, New York, 1974.

Fink M, Klein D F. An ethical dilemma in child psychiatry. *Psychiatric Bull* 1995; 19: 650–1.

Fink M, Sackeim H A. ECT for schizophrenia? *Schizophrenia Bull* 1996; 22: 27–39.

Fink M, Sackeim H A. Theophylline and ECT. *Convulsive Ther* 1998; 14: 286–90.

Fink M, Shaw R, Gross G, et al. Comparative study of chlorpromazine and insulin coma in the therapy of psychosis. *Journal of American Medical Association* 1958; 166: 1846–50.

Fink M, Taylor M A: Catatonia: A separate category for DSM-TV? *Integ Psych* 1991; 7: 2–10.

Fink M, Zervas I M. ECT and delirium in Parkinson's disease. Letter. *J Neuropsychiatry Clin Neurosci* 1992; 4: 231–2.

Flach F. *Rickie.* 275 pp. Fawcett Columbine, New York, 1990.

Flint A J, Rifat S L. Two-year outcome of psychotic depression in late life. *Am J Psychiatry* 1998; 155: 178–83.

Foucault M. *Madness and Civilization.* Translated by R. Howard. New American Library, New York, 1965.

Frankel F H. Electro-convulsive therapy in Massachusetts: A task force report. *Mass Jrl Mental Hlth* 1973; 3: 3–29.

Freeman H. *Judge, Jury and Executioner.* Talking Leaves Publishing Co., Urbana, Illinois, 1986.

Fricchione G L, Kaufman L D, Gruber B L, Fink M. Electroconvulsive therapy and cyclophosphamide in combination for severe neuropsychiatric lupus with catatonia. *Am J Medicine* 1990; 88: 443–4.

Gelenberg A J: The catatonic syndrome. *Lancet* 1976; 2: 1339–41.

Gelenberg A J, Mandel M R. Catatonic reactions to high-potency neuroleptic drugs. *Arch Gen Psychiatry* 1977; 34: 947–50.

Geoghegan J J, Stevenson G H. Prophylactic electroshock. *Am J Psychiatry* 1949; 105: 494–6.

Ghaziuddin N. Use of electroconvulsive therapy in childhood psychiatric disorders. *Child Adolesc Psychopharm News* 1998; 3: 1–8.

Gilbert D A, Altshuler K Z, Rabo W V et al. Texas Medication Algorithm Project: Definitions, rationale, and methods to develop medication algorithms. *J Clin Psychiatry* 1998; 59: 345–51.

Glassman A H, Kantor S J, Shostak M. Depression, delusions, and drug response. *Am J Psychiatry* 1975; 132: 716–9.

Gotkin J, Gotkin P. *Too Much Anger, Too Much Tears: A Personal Triumph Over Psychiatry.* Quadrangle/The New York Times Book Co., New York, 1975.

Graham K. *Personal History.* Knopf, New York, 1997a. Also as audiotape read by the author, published by Random House Audio Publishing Inc., 1997b.

Graham P J, Foreman D M. An ethical dilemma in child and adolescent psychiatry. *Psychiatric Bull* 1995; 19: 84–6.

Green A I, Zalma A, Berman I, et al. Clozapine following ECT: A two-step treatment. *J Clin Psychiatry* 1994; 55(9): 388–90.

Greenberg L B, Anand A., Roque C T, et al. Electroconvulsive therapy and cerebral venous angioma. *Convulsive Ther* 1986; 2: 197–202.

Greenberg L B, Fink M. Electroconvulsive therapy in the elderly. *Psychiatric Annals* 1990; 20: 99–101.

Greenberg L B, Gujavarty K. The neuroleptic malignant syndrome: Review and report of three cases. *Comprehens Psychiatry* 1985; 26: 63–70.

Greenberg L B, Mofson R, Fink M. Prospective electroconvulsive therapy in a delusional depressed patient with a frontal meningioma. *Br J Psychiatry* 1988; 153: 105–7.

Griesemer D A, Kellner C H, Beale M D, et al. Electroconvulsive therapy for treatment of intractable seizures. Initial findings in two children. *Neurology* 1997; 49: 1389–92.

Grob G. *The Inner World of American Psychiatry 1890–1940: Selected Correspondence.* Rutgers University Press, New Brunswick, NJ, 1985.

Grob G. *The Mad Among Us.* 386 pp. Free Press, New York, 1994.

Grosser G H, Pearsall D T, Fisher C L, et al. The regulation of electroconvulsive treatment in Massachusetts: A follow-up. *Mass Jrl Mental Hlth* 1975; 5: 12–24.

Group for the Advancement of Psychiatry (GAP). *Shock Therapy.* Report No. 1. Topeka, K S. (Quoted in full in Fink, 1979, p. 14.)

Grunhaus L. *Electroconvulsive Therapy (ECT). The Treatment, the Questions and the Answers.* Informational videotape. MECTA Corporation, Lake Oswego, OR, 1988.

Guinier L. *Lift Every Voice.* Simon & Schuster, 1998, p. 119.

Gujavarty K, Greenberg L B, Fink M. Electroconvulsive therapy and neuroleptic medication in the treatment of therapy resistant positive-symptom psychosis. *Convulsive Ther* 1987; 3: 111–20.

Gurevitz S, Helme W H. Effects of electroconvulsive therapy on personality and intellectual functioning of the schizophrenic child. *J Nerv Ment Dis* 120: 213–26, 1954.

Guttmacher L B, Cretella H. Electroconvulsive therapy in one child and three adolescents. *J Clin Psychiatry* 1988; 49: 20–3.

Hasan S, Buckley P. Novel antipsychotics and the neuroleptic malignant syndrome: A review and critique. *Am J Psychiatry* 1998; 155: 1113–6.

Hermann R C, Dorwart R A, Hoover C W, et al. Variation in ECT use in the United States. *Am J Psychiatry* 1995; 152: 869–75.

Hermann R C, Ettner S, Dorwart R A, et al. Characteristics of psychiatrists who perform ECT. *Am J Psychiatry* 1998; 155: 889–94.

Hoch A. *Benign Stupors.* Macmillan, New York, 1921.

Holmberg G. The factor of hypoxemia in electroshock therapy. *Am J Psychiatry* 1953a; 110: 115–18.

Holmberg G. The influence of oxygen administration on electrically induced convulsions in man. *Acta Psychiatr Neurol* 1953b; 28: 365–86.

Holmberg G, Thesleff S. Succinylcholine-iodide as a muscular relaxant in electroshock therapy. *Am J Psychiatry* 1952; 108: 842–6.

Isaac R J, Armat V C. *Madness in the Streets: How Psychiatry and the Law Abandoned the Mentally Ill.* 436 pp. Free Press, New York, 1990.

Janis I L. Memory loss following electric convulsive treatments. *J Personality* 1948; 17: 29–32.

Janis I L. Psychological effects of electric convulsive treatments (posttreatment amnesias). *J Nerv Ment Dis* 1950; 111: 359–82.

Jessner L, Ryan V G. *Shock Treatment in Psychiatry: A Manual.* 149 pp. Grune & Stratton, New York, 1941.

Kahlbaum K L: *Catatonia.* Johns Hopkins University Press, Baltimore, 1973.

Kalinowsky L B, Kennedy F. Observations in electric shock therapy applied to problems of epilepsy. *J Nerv Ment Dis* 1943; 98: 56–67.

Kane J M, Honigfeld G, Singer J, et al. Clozapine for the treatment-resistant schizophrenic. *Arch Gen Psychiatry* 1988; 45: 789–96.

Kane J M, McGlashan T H. Treatment of schizophrenia. *Lancet* 1995; 346: 820–5.

Kane J M, Smith J M. Tardive dyskinesia: Prevalence and risk factors, 1959–1979. *Arch Gen Psychiatry* 1982; 39: 473–81.

Kane J M, Woerner M, Weinhold P, et al. Incidence of tardive dyskinesia: Five-year data from a prospective study. *Psychopharmacol Bull* 1984; 20: 387–9.

Kantor S J, Glassman A H. Delusional depressions: Natural history and response to treatment. *Br J Psychiatry* 1977; 131: 351–60.

Karliner W, Wehrheim H K. Maintenance convulsive treatments. *Am J Psychiatry* 1965; 121: 113–5.

Katzenelbogen S, Santee F. The treatment of schizophrenia: Insulin shock. Cardiozol. Sleep treatment. *Am J Psychiatry* 1938; 94: Supplement 1–354. American Psychiatric Association, Washington, D.C.

Keisling R. Successful treatment of an unidentified patient with one ECT. *Am J Psychiatry* 1984; 141: 148.

Kellner C H (ed). *Electroconvulsive Therapy. Psychiatric Clinics NA.* 14: 793–1035, 1991.

Kellner C H, Fink M. Seizure adequacy: Does EEG hold the key? *Convulsive Ther* 1996; 12: 203–6.

Kiloh L G. Pseudo-dementia. *Acta Psychiatr Scand* 1961; 37: 336–51.

King B H, Liston E H. Proposals for the mechanism of action of convulsive therapy: A synthesis. *Biol Psychiatry* 1990; 27: 76–94.

Klaesi J. Über die therapeutische Anwendung der "Dauernarkose" mittels Somnifen bei Schizophrenen. *Ztschr f d ges Psychiat u Neurol* 1922; 74: 557–67.

Klapheke M M. Combining ECT and antipsychotic agents: Benefits and risks. *Convulsive Ther* 1989; 9: 241–55.

Klerman G. The psychiatric patient's right to effective treatment: Implications of Osheroff v. Chestnut Lodge. *Am J Psychiatry* 1990; 147: 409–18.

Kramer B A. Use of ECT in California, 1977–1983. *Am J Psychiatry* 1985; 142: 1190–2.

Kramer B A. Use of ECT in California, revisited: 1984–1994. *Am J Psychiatry* (in press).

Kroessler D. Relative efficacy rates for therapies of delusional depression. *Convulsive Ther* 1985; 1: 173–82.

Krystal A D, Watts B V, Weiner R D, et al. The use of flumazenil in the anxious and benzodiazepine-dependent ECT patient. *JECT* 1998; 14: 5–14.

LaGrone D. ECT in secondary mania, pregnancy, and sickle cell anemia. *Convulsive Ther* 1990; 6 176–80.

Landy D A. Combined use of clozapine and electroconvulsive therapy. *Convulsive Ther* 1991; 7: 218–21.

Lask B, Britten C, Kroll L, et al. Children with pervasive refusal. *Arch Dis Childhood* 1991; 66: 866–9.

Latey R H, Fahy T J. *Electroconvulsive Therapy in the Republic of Ireland. 1982.* Galway University Press, Galway, 1982.

Lazarus A, Mann S C, Caroff S N. *The Neuroleptic Malignant Syndrome and Related Conditions.* 268 pp. American Psychiatric Press, Washington D.C., 1989.

Lebensohn Z M. Electroconvulsive therapy: Psychiatry's villain or hero? *Am Jrl Social Psychiatry* 1984; 4:39–43.

Lebensohn Z M, Jenkins R B. Improvement of parkinsonism in depressed patients treated with ECT. *Am J Psychiatry* 1975; 132: 283–5.

Lerer B, Shapira B, Calev A, et al. Antidepressant and cognitive effects of twice-versus three-times-weekly ECT. *Am J Psychiatry* 1995; 152: 564–70.

Lowenstein D H, Alldredge B K. Status epilepticus. *NEJM* 1998; 338: 970–6.

Maletzky B M. *Multiple-Monitored Electroconvulsive Therapy.* 238 pp. , CRC Press, Boca Raton, FL, 1981.

Malitz S, Sackeim H A (eds). *Electroconvulsive Therapy: Clinical and Basic Research Issues.* NY Acad Sci 1986; 462: 1–424.

Manning M. *Undercurrents: A Therapist's Reckoning with Depression.* Harper-Collins, New York, 1994.

Markowitz J, Brown R, Sweeney J, et al. Reduced length and cost of hospital stay for major depression in patients treated with ECT. *Am J Psychiatry* 1987; 144: 1025–9.

McCall W V, Mann S C, Shelp F E, Caroff S N. Fatal pulmonary embolism in the catatonic syndrome. Two case reports and a literature review. *J Clin Psychiatry* 1995; 56: 21–5.

McEvoy J P, et al. Treatment of schizophrenia: Expert consensus guideline. *J Clin Psychiatry* 1996; 57: Supplement 12B, 1–58.

MECTA Corporation. *Electroconvulsive Therapy (ECT): The treatment, the questions and the answers.* Information booklet. MECTA Corporation, 1988.

Meduna L. Versuche über die biologische Beeinflussung des Ablaufes der Schizophrenie: Camphor und Cardiozolkrampfe. *Z ges Neurol Psychiatr* 1935; 152: 235–62.

Meduna L. *Die Konvulsionstherapie der Schizophrenie.* Karl Marhold, Halle a. S., 1937. pp. 121.

Meduna L. *Carbon Dioxide Therapy.* 236 pp. Charles C Thomas, Springfield, IL., 1950a.

Meduna L. *Oneirophrenia.* University of Illinois Press, Urbana, 1950b.

Meduna L. Autobiography. *Convulsive Ther* 1985; 1: 43–57, 121–38.

Miller M C. ECT and mania. *Am J Psychiatry* 1995; 152: 654.

Mitchell P, Hadzi-Pavlovic D, Parker G, et al. Depressive psychomotor disturbance, cortisol, and dexamethasone. *Biol Psychiatry* 1996; 40: 941–50.

Moise F N, Petrides G. Case study: Electroconvulsive therapy in adolescents. *J Am Acad Child Adolesc Psychiatry* 1996; 35: 312–18.

Moore N P. The maintenance treatment of chronic psychotics by electrically induced convulsions. *J Ment Sci* 1943; 89: 257–69.

Mukherjee S, Sackeim H A, Schnur D B. Electroconvulsive therapy of acute manic episodes: A review of 50 years' experience. *Am J Psychiatry* 1994; 151: 169–76.

Mulsant B H, Haskett R F, Prudic J, et al. Low use of neuroleptic drugs in the treatment of psychotic major depression. *Am J Psychiatry* 1997; 154: 559–61.

Murillo L G, Exner J E. The effects of regressive ECT with process schizophrenics. *Am J Psychiatry* 1973; 130: 269–73.

Myers B S, Kalayam B, Mei-Tal V. Late-onset delusional depression: A distinct clinical entity? *J Clin Psychiatry* 1984; 45: 347–9.

Myers B S, Kalayam B, Mei-Tal V. Delusional depression in the elderly. In C A Shamoian (ed), *Treatment of Affective Disorders in the Elderly,* pp. 19–28. American Psychiatric Association Press, Washington, D.C. 1985.

Nelson J C, Davis J M. DST studies in psychotic depression. A meta-analysis. *Am J Psychiatry* 1997; 154: 1497–1503.

Nemeroff C B, Bissette G, Akil H, Fink M. Neuropeptide concentrations in the cerebrospinal fluid of depressed patients treated with electroconvulsive therapy: Corticotrophin-releasing factor, beta-endorphin and somatostatin. *Br J Psychiatry* 1991; 158: 59–63.

News and Notes, *Convulsive Ther* 1992; 8: 221–2; and 1993; 9: 69–73.

Nobler M S, Sackeim H A. Augmentation strategies in electroconvulsive therapy: A synthesis. *Convulsive Ther* 1993; 9: 331–51.

Nutt D J. Not only but also? *Neuropsychopharm* 1990; 3: 93–5.

Olfson M, Marcus S, Sackeim H A, et al. Use of ECT for the inpatient treatment of recurrent major depression. *Am J Psychiatry* 1998; 155: 22–9.

Papolos D, Papolos J. *Overcoming Depression.* Third Ed. HarperPerennial, New York, 1997.

Parry B L. The tragedy of legal impediments involved in obtaining ECT for patients unable to give informed consent. Letter. *Am J Psychiatry* 1981; 138: 1128–9.

Petrides G. Continuation ECT: A review. *Annals Clin Psychiatry* (in press).

Petrides G, Dhosshe D, Fink M, et al. Continuation ECT: Relapse prevention in affective disorders. *Convulsive Ther* 1994; 10: 189–94.

Petrides G, Fink M. Atrial fibrillation, anticoagulation, and electroconvulsive therapy. *Convulsive Ther* 1996a; 12: 91–8.

Petrides G, Fink M. The "half-age" stimulation strategy for ECT dosing. *Convulsive Ther* 1996b; 12: 138–46.

Philibert R A, Richards L, Lynch C F, et al. Effect of ECT on mortality and clinical outcome in geriatric unipolar depression. *J Clin Psychiatry* 1995; 56: 390–4.

Pippard J. Audit of electroconvulsive treatment in two national health service regions. *Br J Psychiatry* 1992; 160: 621–37.

Pippard J, Ellam L. *Electroconvulsive Therapy in Great Britain, 1980.* 108 pp. Gaskell, London, 1981.

Plath S. *The Bell Jar.* Harper & Row, New York, 1971.

Post R. ECT: The anticonvulsant connection. *Neuropsychopharm* 1990; 3: 89–92.

Powell J C, Silviera W R, Lindsay R. Pre-pubertal depressive stupor: A case report. *Br J Psychiatry* 1988; 153: 689–92.

A Practicing Psychiatrist. The experience of electro-convulsive therapy. *Br J Psychiatry* 1965; 111: 365–7.

Prien R F, Kupfer D J. Continuation drug therapy in the prevention of recurrences in unipolar and bipolar affective disorders. *Am J Psychiatry* 1986; 143: 18–23.

Prudic J, Sackeim H A, Devanand D, et al. Medication resistance and clinical response to electroconvulsive therapy. *Psychiatry Res* 1990; 31: 287–96.

Rasmussen K, Abrams R. Treatment of Parkinson's disease with electroconvulsive therapy. *Psych Clin North Am* 1991; 14: 925–33.

Reid W H, Keller S, Leatherman M, et al. ECT in Texas: 19 months of mandatory reporting. *J Clin Psychiatry* 1998; 59: 8–13.

Rey J M, Walter G. Half a century of ECT use in young people. *Am J Psychiatry* 154: 595–602, 1997.

Rich C L. Recovery from depression after one ECT. *Am J Psychiatry* 1984; 141: 1010-1.

Röder T, Kubillus V, Burwell A. *Psychiatrists—The Men Behind Hitler.* Freedom Publishing, Los Angeles, 1995.

Rodger C R, Scott A I F, Whalley L J. Is there a delay in the onset of the antidepressant effect of electroconvulsive therapy? *Br J Psychiatry* 1994; 164: 106–9.

Rorsman B, Hagnell O, Lauke J. Psychiatric mortality in the Lundby study: An overview. *Acta Psychiatr Belg* 1986; 42: 98–103.

Rouechè B. As Empty as Eve. *The New Yorker*, Sept. 9, 1974, pp. 84–100.

Royal College of Psychiatrists. *The Official Video Teaching Pack.* 1994. London, UK.

Roy-Byrne P, Gerner R H. Legal restrictions on the use of ECT in California: Clinical impact on the incompetent patient. *J Clin Psychiatry* 1981; 42: 300–3.

Rush A J, Giles D E, Schlesser M A, et al. The dexamethasone suppression test in patients with mood disorders. *J Clin Psychiatry* 1996; 57: 470–84.

Sackeim H A (ed). Mechanisms of action. *Convulsive Ther* 1989; 5: 207–304.

Sackeim H A. Are ECT devices underpowered? *Convulsive Ther* 1991; 7: 233–6.

Sackeim H A. The cognitive effects of electroconvulsive therapy. In W H Moos, E R Gamzu, L J Thal (eds), *Cognitive disorders: pathophysiology and treatment,* pp. 183–228. Marcel Dekker, New York, 1992.

Sackeim H A, Decina P, Portnoy S, et al. Studies of dosage, seizure threshold, and seizure duration in ECT. *Biol Psychiatry* 1987; 22: 249–68.

Sackeim H A, Decina P, Prohovnik I, et al. Anticonvulsant and antidepressant properties of electroconvulsive therapy: A proposed mechanism of action. *Biol Psychiatry* 1983; 18: 1301–10.

Sackeim H A, Devenand D. Why we do not know how convulsive therapy works. *Neuropsychopharm* 1990; 3: 83–7.

Sackeim H A, Luber B, Katzman G P, et al. The effects of electroconvulsive therapy on quantitative electroencephalograms. *Arch Gen Psychiatry* 1996; 53: 814–24.

Sackeim H A, Prudic J, Devanand D P, et al. The impact of medication resistance and continuation pharmacotherapy on relapse following response to electroconvulsive therapy in major depression. *J Clin Psychopharmacol* 1990; 10: 96–104.

Sackeim H A, Prudic, J, Devanand D, et al. Effects of stimulus intensity and electrode placement on the efficacy and cognitive effects of electroconvulsive therapy. *N Engl J Med* 1993; 328: 839–46.

Safferman A Z, Munne R. Combining clozapine with ECT. Case report. *Convulsive Ther* 1992; 8: 141–3.

Sargent M. *Depressive Disorders: Treatments Bring New Hope.* US DHEW 86-1491, NIMH, Rockville, MD. Information booklet. 9 pp., 1986.

Sattin A. The role of TRH and related peptides in the mechanism of action of ECT. *JECT* 1999; 15: 76–92.

Schatzberg A F, Rothschild A J. Psychotic (delusional) major depression: should it be included as a distinct syndrome in DSM-IV? *Am J Psychiatry,* 1993; 149: 733–45.

Schneekloth T D, Rummans T A, Logan K M. Electroconvulsive therapy in adolescents. *Convulsive Ther* 1993; 9: 158–66.

Schnur D B, Mukherjee S, Silver J, et al. Electroconvulsive therapy in the treatment of episodic aggressive dyscontrol in psychotic patients. *Convulsive Ther* 1989; 5: 353–61.

Schönbauer L, Jantsch M. *Julius Wagner-Jauregg: Lebenserrinerungen.* 187 pp. Springer-Verlag, Vienna, 1950.

Shorter E. *A History of Psychiatry.* John Wiley & Sons, New York, 1997.

Shutts D. *Lobotomy: Resort to the Knife.* 284 pp. Van Nostrand Reinhold Co., New York, 1982,

Singer E, Garfinkel R, Cohen S M, et al. Mortality and mental health: Evidence from the Midtown Manhattan Restudy. *Soc Sci Med* 1976; 10: 517–25.

Solomon A. Anatomy of melancholy. *The New Yorker,* Jan. 12, 1998, pp. 46–64.

Spock B. *The Common Sense Book of Baby and Child Care.* Duell, Sloan & Pearce, New York, 1946.

Spock B. *Baby and Child Care,* Pocket Books, New York, 1957, 1968, 1976, 1985, 1992.

Squire S. Shock therapy's return to respectability: Once the subject of horror stories, ECT is receiving new acceptance as a valuable psychiatric tool. *NY Times Magazine,* Nov. 22, 1987, pp. 78–79, 85, 88–9.

Steir C. *Blue Jolts.* New Republic Books, Washington, D.C. 1978.

Steffens D C, Krystal A D, Sibert T E, et al. Cost effectiveness of maintenance ECT. *Convulsive Ther* 1995; 11: 283–4.

Stevenson G H, Geoghegan J J. Prophylactic electroshock. *Am J Psychiatry* 1951; 107: 743–8.

Stone G. Short sharp shocks. *New York* 1994, pp. 55–9.

Straus E. *Roslyn Yalow, Nobel Laureate.* Plenum Press, New York, 1998.

Styron, W. *Darkness Visible.* 85 pp. New York, Random House, 1990.

Swartz C M. Double stimulation can bypass safety standards. *Convulsive Ther* 1991; 7: 302–3.

Swartz C M, Mehta R K. Double electroconvulsive therapy for resistant depression. *Convulsive Ther* 1986; 2:55–7.

Szasz T S. *The Myth of Mental Illness. Foundations of a Theory of Personal Conduct.* 337 pp. Paul B. Hoeber Co., New York, 1961.

Taylor M A. Catatonia: A review of the behavioral neurologic syndrome. *Neuropsychiat, Neuropsychol & Behav Neurol* 1990; 3: 48–72.

Taylor M A, Abrams R. The phenomenology of mania: A new look at some old patients. *Arch Gen Psychiatry* 1973; 29: 520–2.

Taylor M A, Abrams R. Catatonia: Prevalence and importance in the manic phase of manic-depressive illness. *Arch Gen Psychiatry* 1977; 34: 1223–5.

Terry G C. *Fever and Psychoses.* 167 pp. Paul B. Hoeber, New York, 1939.

Thompson J W, Weiner R D, Mayers C P. Use of ECT in the United States in 1975, 1980, 1986. *Am J Psychiatry* 1994; 151: 1657–61.

Thuppal M, Fink M. Electroconvulsive therapy and mental retardation. *JECT* (in press).

Tomson T, Lindbom U, Nilsson B Y, et al. Serum prolactin during status epilepticus. *J Neurol Neurosurg Psychiatry* 1989; 52: 1435–7.

Trezise K. Changes in practice of ECT: a follow-on study. *Psychiatric Bull* 1998; 22: 687–90.

Trimble M. Serum prolactin in epilepsy and hysteria. *BMJ* 1978; 2: 1682.

Usdin E, Hamburg D A, Barchas J D (ed). *Neuroregulators and Psychiatric Disorders.* 627 pp. Oxford University Press, New York, 1977.

Wagner-Jauregg J. Über die Einwirkung der Malaria auf die Progressive Paralyse. *Psychiatr-Neurol Wchnschr* 1918; 20: 132–51.

Walter G, Rey J M. An epidemiological study of the use of ECT in adolescents. *J Am Acad Child Adolesc Psychiatry* 1997; 36: 809–15.

Weigert E. Psychoanalytic notes on sleep and convulsion treatment in functional psychoses. *Psychiatry* 1940; 3: 189–209.

Weinstein E A, Kahn R L. *Denial of Illness.* 166 pp. Charles C Thomas, Springfield, IL., 1955.

Viparelli U, Viparelli G. ECT and grand-mal epilepsy. *Convulsive Ther* 1992; 8: 39–42.

Vonnegut M. *The Eden Express: A Personal Account of Schizophrenia.* Praeger Publishers, New York, 1975.

Woerner M G, Alvir J M, Saltz B L, et al. Prospective study of tardive dyskinesia in the elderly: Rates and risk factors. *Am J Psychiatry* 1998; 155: 1521–28.

Working Group on Status Epilepticus. Treatment of status epilepticus. *JAMA* 1993; 270: 854–9.

Wyatt R J. Neuroleptics and the natural course of schizophrenia. *Schizophrenia Bull* 1991; 17: 325–51.

Wyden P. *Conquering Schizophrenia.* 335 pp. Knopf, New York, 1998.

Zervas I M, Fink M. ECT for refractory Parkinson's disease. *Convulsive Ther* 1991; 7: 222–3.

Index

APACK

11/99

8648